Naturopathic Basic Science
Board Review
Study Questions

Naturopathic Basic Science Board Review Study Questions

2013 Edition

Kathryn Yash, BA, ND

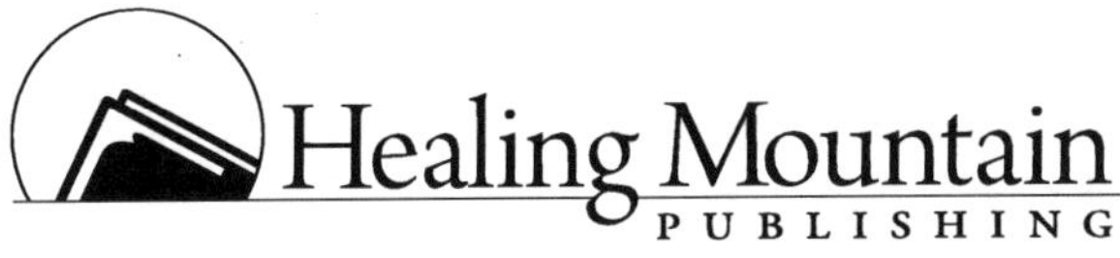

Healing Mountain PUBLISHING

Seattle   Wenatchee

DISCLAIMER

The information provided in this study manual is not sanctioned or approved by the Naturopathic Physicians Licensing Exam (NPLEX) or North American Board of Naturopathic Examiners (NABNE). This manual is not published or distributed by NPLEX, NABNE, or any of its representatives. It was created by the authors and published by Healing Mountain Publishing independent of NPLEX and NABNE solely for educational purposes. In no way is NPLEX or NABNE accountable for the content of this guide. The NPLEX/NABNE blueprint included in its official study guide is the copyrighted property of NPLEX and thus cannot be included in this manual.

Note that the NPLEX/NABNE blueprint is not definitive about the content of the NPLEX/NABNE board examinations. In many cases it does not give a complete listing of examination content, which means that anything included in a topic area can be the basis of examination questions. For this reason, the study manual itself cannot be definitive and serves mainly to expand points noted in the blueprint, leaving more detailed study and exploration of the sections to the student.

While new additions are being added to the NPLEX/NABNE blueprint throughout the year, the manual is updated only once during that time. The authors have no control over changes in the NPLEX/NABNE blueprint and do not guarantee that this manual will cover last-minute changes to the blueprint prior to the date of the examination. For this reason, we do not recommend that you purchase this manual prior to the year in which you plan to sit for the board examinations. If you have any questions in this regard, you can contact NPLEX/NABNE to determine if any significant modifications to the blueprint were made in a given year. We highly recommend that you purchase the latest blueprint prior to sitting for the examinations.

The information contained in this guide is purely for educational purposes. It is not intended to take the place of medical care and is not designed as a comprehensive clinical reference. As medicine is an ever-changing field, the information in this guide can become out-of-date.

Healing Mountain Publishing, Inc.
430 Elva Wy
E Wenatchee, WA 98802

(888) 405-8727

www.healingmountainpublishing.com

Book design and typesetting by Dave Howell. Set in Adobe Jensen.
Cover by Brad Fitzgerald.

ISBN: 978-1-933350-75-2

Contents

Author Bio

Kathryn Yash, BA, ND

Growing up in a family of nurses, doctors, and herbalists meant that Dr. Yash was destined for the healthcare field. After pursuing a bachelor's in contemplative psychology with honours, Dr. Yash moved on to the Canadian College of Naturopathic Medicine (CCNM) to pursue her passion of naturopathic medicine. While at CCNM, Dr. Yash volunteered her time with the Ontario Association of Naturopathic Doctors and the Naturopathic Students Association. Her contributions in those areas and as a class representation resulted in the 2010 Naturopathic Honour Award. Her future aspirations are to develop a successful general care practice, become a certified meditation instructor, and undergo further training in endocrinology and neurology.

Introduction

Congratulations on getting to the half way point in your Naturopathic Medical Training! The Biomedical Science Exam is the next hurdle before you begin your clinical years. One thing that has not changed over the years, is the need to know your stuff when taking NPLEX exams.

The purpose of this book is to offer you another tool to review and deepen your knowledge when studying for the Biomedical Science Exam. The publishers and I have attempted to make this book as helpful as possible by changing the sections to reflex those in the NABNE Study Guide, adding in new multiple choice questions, and reviewing all the questions to ensure they are accurate and un-ambiguous. If you come across an inaccurate question, then please don't hesitate to contact us.

Multiple Choice Questions

Time and again, what students find the most helpful when studying for the Basic Science Exam are practice exams. At the end of this book, you will find some multiple choice questions that will help test your knowledge. These questions are by no means exhaustive, given the vast scope of material that NABNE expects students to know. I trust you will find these test questions helpful. Don't stress over getting a question wrong. Just think of missed questions as a guide for what you need to review a little more.

This Book and NABNE

These questions are not produced by NABNE. They are neither published, endorsed, nor distributed by NABNE. This book is for educational purposes and is a study aid. These questions follow the NABNE Study Guide as closely as possible and represent a wide range of possible questions that may appear on the examination. Unfortunately due to page limitation and changing curriculum, this book cannot cover all the areas that NABNE expects you to be proficient in.

Also, It is important to remember that the Board exams often have questions that are not covered in the NABNE Study Guide. The Study Guide serves only as a blueprint to what areas may appear on the exam. It provides a topic and a list of competencies— it does not provide a complete list of examples. Anything included in a topic area is fair game for testing. Be warned that NABNE doesn't just test on broad concepts, but rather tends to focus on nit-picky details.

How the Questions Were Written

The original author of this book came up with the initial questions while he was studying. He tried to figure out how the folks at NABNE would ask questions of the material he was reading. For instance:

INFORMATION FROM PHYSIOLOGY TEXTBOOK:

Carbohydrates are found in the cell membrane and function as cell-to-cell communicators.

POTENTIAL NPLEX QUESTION:

What mediates cell-to-cell communication in the cell membrane? *Carbohydrates*

Illegal Copying

Please do not make photocopies of this manual or buy it second hand. This manual was produced by a fellow naturopathic physician and a future colleague of yours. It took many hours to produce this book and takes many hours every year to update it. It is not a perfect study tool, but the effort is made every year with the goal of helping out the Naturopathic community during a very stressful and important time in their education.

The prices are very reasonable. The prices are set with the aim of recouping the cost of printing the books and the time it takes to coordinate that effort. The less books that are bought the greater the price increase, because printers charge higher rates as the volume of books produced lessens. Meaning the less people who buy the book, the more expensive the book becomes and the less resources there are for updating and editing the book. Healing Mountain Publishing is a small, 3 person, on the side, job and not some large multi-national conglomerate out to eat up all your money. If you feel as though the prices are unreasonable and have ideas for how to adjust that, then by all means contact us and share them.

Recent Updates

Over the past few years, I've gone back through and edited the questions composed by the previous author with the goal of removing erroneous questions. Also, I've done the tedious task of going through the book question by question to ensure that the general competencies expected by NABNE are covered. Where there was a gap between what the book covered and what the NABNE Study Guide expected, I added in questions on the matter. Unfortunately, there is no way to cover everything you need to know for the exam. Think of this book as a good starting place for reviewing what you've already studied.

Thanks to students who took the time to give feedback, many of the grammatical errors and inconsistencies have been fixed. Sadly something always gets missed when correcting these items, so if you happen to notice any mistakes, then please contact us. Whether it is grammatical or technical in nature, please let Healing Mountain Publishing know. As well as, we always welcome any suggestion you have for making the books into better study tools. We love and invite constructive student feedback on any aspects of any of the books.

Abbreviations

In order to save space the following common abbreviations exist throughout the book:

ACTH = Adrenocorticotropin hormone ADH = Antidiuretic hormone DHEA = Dehydropiondrosterone DHT = Dihydrotestosterone EFA = Essential fatty acids Epi = Epinephrine FA = Fatty Acid FSH = Follicle stimulating hormone G.I. = Gastrointestinal tract GH = Growth hormone GHRH = Growth hormone releasing hormone GNRH = Gonadotropin releasing hormone HCL = Hydrochloric acid HDL = High-density lipoprotein IGFS = Insulin-like growth factors LDL = Low-density lipoprotein LH = Luteinizing hormone L.I. = Large intestine K = Potassium NA = Sodium Norepi = Norepinephrine PRH = Prolactin releasing hormone PTH = Parathyroid hormone S.I. = Small intestine TRH = Thyroid releasing hormone TSH = Thyroid stimulating hormone VLDL = Very low-density lipoprotein

Study Strategies And Tips

How to Use This Book

At the front of the *Naturopathic Basic Science Boards Study Manual* published by Healing Mountain Publishing is an excellent section on study skills. If you have not read that section I highly recommend that you do because there are some tools in there that will help you pass this exam.

People have asked me how this book works with *Naturopathic Basic Science Boards Study Manual*. This book's sole aim is to help you recall information that is stored inside your brain. Over the last couple of years you have been absorbed in naturopathic medicine. In that time you have been tested over and over again so hopefully by now the information has become part of you. My aim is to bring a lot of that knowledge to the surface so when you sit down in front of your multiple choice examination the correct answer is very easy to identify.

I recommend that you thoroughly study the *Naturopathic Basic Science Boards Study Guide*. Become very familiar with the material and then use this book as a way to test whether or not you know the facts. Go through the cases at the back of this book towards the end of your study period.

I recommend covering up the answers on the right hand side and going down the list of questions to test yourself. Also get together with a group of friends during the last week of studying and test each other over and over again. This technique of studying is a wonderful way to see what you know and what you do not know.

Brain Waves and Studying

When I studied for my boards I did some research online to identify the best states to be in to maximize the time spent studying. This research led me to some interesting information about the different brain wave frequencies.

There are 4 brain wave patterns: Alpha, Beta, Delta, and Theta waves.

ALPHA Alpha wave states are associated with a slowing of brain activity and relaxation. You will be more focused when you are in Alpha while remaining relaxed. Some have called Alpha the 'super-learning' state.

BETA The beta brain wave pattern is the pattern of normal waking consciousness and has the most rapid frequency. Beta is associated with concentration, arousal, alertness, and cognition.

DELTA The slowest brain wave pattern is delta, the brain wave pattern of dreamless sleep.

THETA The Theta state is slower than Alpha and is the state the brain is when in dreaming sleep. Don't be put off by Theta because it is also associated with a number of other beneficial states, including increased creativity, some kinds of "super learning," increased memory abilities, and what are called integrative experiences. Interestingly enough the Theta state is the state you should try to get in to during your study periods.

Studying Routine

It is important that you establish a regular study routine. I have included below some of the techniques I used to help pass my exams and to get me into the Theta Wave State.

Exercise

15–60 minutes of aerobic exercise per day

10–30 minutes of anaerobic exercises:

    30 second sprints

    3–5 minute anaerobic pushes

        Climb stairs

        Walk or run up hill

        Power walk around block

        Couple of minutes of squats or push-ups

Benefits:

↑ Oxygen to brain

↑ Negative ions

↑ Glucose and other nutrients to brain

Diet and Nutrition

When you are studying your brain requires a high level of good quality nutrition. I treated my studying periods as if I were training for a marathon. The following are some suggestions for keeping your brain topped up with the best nutrition possible.

Fish, nuts and seeds

Complex carbohydrates and low glycemic index foods

Brain nutrients:

    Minerals: magnesium, Boron, zinc, manganese, chromium and potassium

    Ginseng and Vitamin E to help blood carry oxygen to brain

    Ginkgo to ↑ blood flow to brain

    Antioxidants

    Phosphatidyl choline to ↑ brainpower boosting neurotransmitters

    Amino acids: glutamine, tyrosine and phenylalanine

    Vitamins: B1, 3,6,12, Vitamin C and E

    Others: Acetyl-L-carnitine, DMAE, Spirulina

Brain Smoothies:

    Powdered phosphotidylcholine (PC-55 from Twin Lab)

    Teaspoon of Vitamin C

    Tablespoon of spirulina

    Brewers yeast

    Juice: pineapple, apple, papaya, cranberry etc.

Brain Breaks and Power Naps

When you feel tired or fogged out do a power-nap for 5–15 minutes. The ideal brain wave state to be in for studying is the Theta Wave. This technique is called "Theta Wave Surfing" and is designed to get your brain into the right state for power studying. I took 4 to 5 power naps when I was studying the Boards and I highly recommend that you use it.

Left brain: SHE-ZOME   **Right brain: AH-HEEM**

Technique

Get into a space where you will not be disturbed. Sit in chair, close eyes and silently repeat your word. Repeat it like a tape on a loop i.e. ShezomeShezomeShezome. Find a speed and rhythm that feels comfortable and relaxing i.e. 1X per second. You should find yourself sinking into a deep, cozy place.

Yoga Postures

Yoga is an excellent way to get your body and brain into the right state for studying. Whenever you feel stiff or tired go Theta Wave Surfing with a Brain Break and follow it up with some yoga.

1. **PRANAYAMA OR CONSCIOUS BREATHING (3 TIMES)**
   Feet apart, hands behind head, opening chest and elbows as wide as possible. Inhale slowly and deeply through nose fully filling the lungs and abdomen. On exhale, bring elbows together, and bend knees slowly bringing elbows to knees. Ending up in a crunched position. Inhale returning to upright position.

2. **LEG RAISES (7 TIMES, BUILDING TO 21)**
   Lie on carpet. Put 2 hands palms down with fingers together under the buttocks to support the lower back. Now raise head, chin to chest and exhale through the mouth. Next raise 2 legs with knees locked into vertical position while you inhale through the nose, returning head to the floor. As you return to base position, lower the straightened legs to floor. Chin returns to chest for exhale. Remember: Chin to chest to exhale. Head back to normal position on the inhale. Use a rhythm- do not relax between raising and lowering of the legs

3. **LEAN BACK (7 TIMES, BUILDING UP EACH DAY)**
   Kneel on the floor- knees apart 6–9 inches. Keep body erect with toes flexed to support you. Place hands on back of the thigh muscles. Begin by bringing chin to chest on exhalation. On inhalation move head and neck backwards at same time arching your spine as far as you can. As you arch your back tighten your buttock muscles and brace arms and hands against the back of your thighs for support. Return to base position.

4. **THE TABLE (3 TIMES)**
   Sit on the floor wit legs straight out in front of you with feet 12–15 inches apart with feet flexed. Trunk of the body is erect with palms on the floor facing forward alongside the hips. Begin by bringing chin to chest to exhale. On inhalation move head and neck backward at the same time raising your body so that knees bend as arms straighten.

As you lift your back, your knees go directly over your feet. The trunk of your body and upper legs will be horizontal to the floor like a table. On return to base position, scoot buttocks back to floor near hands. Inhale is when head and body are thrust into table position.

5. DOWNWARD FACING DOG AND PUSH-UP (7 TIMES)
Get onto all fours and position as if you were to do a push-up. Feet and hands should be 2 feet apart. Toes in flexed position. Begin by letting belly sag to ground. Bring head back for a slow deep inhalation through the nose. As you exhale through the mouth raise your butt in the air bending from hips into an inverted "V" position, bringing chin to chest to complete the exhale. Hold your breath as you comeback to the starting position.
From starting position inhale as you slowly lower chest to the floor. Then do a push-up, slowly exhaling as you return to starting position

6. SAVASANA OR CORPSE POSE

Cardiovascular System

Embryology

What germ layer forms the cardiovascular system?	Mesoderm
What germ layer forms the vessels?	Mesoderm
The linear heart tube formed by the mesoderm starts beating on which day of development?	Its first, which is day 15
The embryonic foramen ovale becomes what after birth?	Fossa ovalis
The embryonic ductus arteriosus becomes what after birth?	Ligamentum arteriosum
What forms the atria?	The separation into right and left of the primative sinuatrium or septum primum
The fusion of the endocardial or atrioventricular cushions posteriorly and anteriorly forms what?	The tricuspid and mitral inlets which become the atrioventricular valves
How do the right and left ventricle become compartmentalized?	There are 2 theories on the development a. Trabeculations appear and grow into muscular structures → coalesce with the endoardial cushions → form a interventricular septum eventually b. At the apex a primordial muscular interventricular ridge grows → fuses with the walls of the ventricles → grows up to the endocardial cushion → forms an interventricular foramen

What does the interventricular foramen result in?	By the end of week 7 it closes resulting in the interventricular septum

Anatomy

In what chamber are the SA and AV nodes?	Right atria
Where does blood from cardiac veins flow?	Through the coronary sinus into the right atrium
How much serous fluid lies between the parietal and visceral layer of the pericardium?	Approximately 10-15 ml or cc
What work together to prevent tricuspid and mitral valves from buckling open?	Chordae tendinae and papillary muscle
When do coronary arteries fill?	During diastole blood backs up and fills up the semilunar valves of the aortic valve, entering coronaries
What forms first heart sound?	Closure of the mitral and tricuspid valves
What forms the second heart sound?	Closure of the aortic and pulmonic valves

Angiology

Where does the subclavian artery turn into the axillary artery?	At the lateral border of first rib
At what level of the spine does the vertebral artery enter the transverse foramen?	C6
What are the 2 sources for blood to the CNS?	The vertebral artery The internal carotid
What does the common carotid ascend the neck with?	Internal jugular vein Vagus nerve
What happens to the common carotid between the hyoid bone and upper thyroid cartilage?	It bifurcates into internal and external carotids

What artery supplies all the visceral, musculoskeletal and dental structures of the head and neck appart from the brain and orbit?	The external carotid artery
What artery supplies the orbit? Where does it come form?	Opthalmic artery that branches off from the internal carotid
What is the terminal branch of the external carotid?	The superficial temporal
What is a major source of blood for deep skull cavity, part of the orbit, teeth, muscles of mastication, and the dura mater?	Maxillary artery
What supplies the anterior part of brain?	The internal carotid
What do the 2 vertebral arteries form?	The basilar artery
What supplies the posterior part of brain?	The basilar artery from the 2 vertebral arteries
What arteries comprise the circle of Willis?	Antertior comminucating Anterior Cerebral (R&L) Internal carotid artery (R&L) Posterior cerebral artery (R&L) Posterior communicating artery (L&R)
What purpose does the circle of Willis serve?	It encircles the pituitary gland and the optic chiasma. It unites the brain's anterior and posterior blood supply, equalizes the 2 hemisphere's blood pressure, and provides alternative routes for blood to reach the brain if a vessel becomes compromised
From what artery does the superior cerebellar branch?	Basilar
What branches off form the vertebral artery?	Posterior and anterior spinal arteries Posterior inferior cerebellar
What branches off from the basilar artery?	Superior cerebellar Anterior and middle inferior cerebellar Labarynthine Pontine
What drains blood from scalp and face?	External jugular

What drains blood from brain, superficial face and neck?	Internal jugular
Which jugular vein joins up with subclavian vein?	External jugular
Where does the Arygos Vein drain?	The superior vena cava
What crosses anterior to the scalene tubercle of the 1st rib?	The subclavian vein
What do internal jugular and subclavian become?	Brachiocephalic vein
What travels superficial to SCM?	External jugular
What structures in the dura mater collect venous blood from the brain?	Sinuses
Where do the sinuses drain to?	The internal jugular vein
What structure drains blood from the brain?	Cavernous sinus
What structure provides collateral blood flow through the head?	The pterygoid plexus
What vein travels on the radial side of the arm?	The cephalic vein
What vein travels on the ulnar side of the arm?	Basilic
What vein crosses the cubital fossa?	Median cubital
The basilic vein joins with what to form the inferior portion of the axillary vein?	The brachial vein
What merge into the popliteal vein?	Anterior and Posterior tibial veins
What veins drain into the popliteal vein?	Ant. and post. tibial veins Small saphenous vein
What does the popliteal vein become?	Femoral vein
What drains into the femoral vein?	Great saphenous vein

What vein travels from the medial foot along the medial calf?	Saphenous vein
What vein begins behind medial malleolus and crosses popliteal fossa?	Small saphenous vein
What forms the portal vein?	Superior mesenteric vein Splenic vein
How does blood drain from the liver?	Via sinusoids into hepatic veins and into the inferior vena cava
What drains the greater curvature of the stomach, spleen and pancreas?	The splenic vein
What drains the transverse and the descending colon, sigmoid and rectum?	Inferior mesenteric vein
Where does the inferior mesenteric vein drain?	Into the splenic vein
What does the superior mesenteric vein drain?	Small intestine, ascending colon
What lymphatic vessel drains the lower extremities?	Cisterna chyli
What does the cisterna chyli flow into?	The thoracic duct
True or False: The upper Left side and the lower right and left side of the body's lymph drains into the Thoracic duct?	True, the upper right side of the body (from lower costal margin up to head)drains into the right lymphatic duct, while the rest drains into the thoracic duct
Where does the lymph of the right upper extremity and right neck flow?	Into the right lymphatic duct
Where does the thoracic duct drain?	Into the left subclavian vein
What makes up central lymphatic tissue?	Bone marrow and thymus
What makes up peripheral lymphoid tissue?	Lymph nodes, peyers patches, appendix, tonsils etc.

Physiology

What serves as a conduit for blood?	Arteries
What blood vessel is involved in nutrient and waste exchange?	Capillaries
What are the 3 typs of capillaries?	Continuous Fenestrated Sinusoidal
What type of capillary excludes proteins and cells from passing through?	Continuous
What type of capillary excludes cells? Where are they found?	Fenestrated. Found in the kidney
What type of capillary allows cells and protein to pass through? Where are they found?	Sinusoidal/discontinuous. Found in liver, bone marrow, spleen
What three layers are found in all blood vessels except capillaries?	a. Tunica intima or interna b. Tunica media c. Tunica adventitia or externa
What property of blood vessels helps push blood through arteriole system?	Elastic tissue
What property of blood vessels does smooth muscle provide?	Its ability to contract and dilate allows blood to be shunted from one area to another
What protects blood vessels against distention?	The fibrous nature of the tissue
Which blood vessel layer contains collagen and elastic fibers?	Tunica adventitia
Capillaries are comprised of only one of these layers; which is it?	Tunica intima
Which blood vessel layer contains smooth muscle and thus is responsible for vasoconstriction and vasodilation?	Tunica Media
What types of blood vessels are resistance vessels due to their smooth muscle?	Arteries and arterioles

Myocardial cells have more of this organelle due to its high oxidative capacity	Mitochondria
What cellular feature allows the heart to contract in unison?	The presence of gap junctions between muscle cells
How do T-tubules differ between cardiac and skeletal muscle cells?	Cardiac: T-tubules contain extracellular fluid high in calcium Skeletal: T-tubules contain extracellular fluid low in calcium
What structure brings depolarization inside the cardiac muscle and helps regulate cytoplasmic calcium?	T tubules
What prevents tetanic contraction in cardiac muscle?	The long cardiac action potential
What aspect of the action potential prevents a second action potential from taking place?	The long refractory period or plateau period
What is the originator of the cardiac action potential?	The SA node
What property allows the SA node to function as the primary pacemaker?	The small size of the cells allow for it to spontaneously depolarize
What acts as a delay station for the action potential?	The AV node
Why does the AV node delay the action potential?	To allow the atrial muscle to depolarize before the ventricular muscle
What can act as a secondary pacemaker in pathological conditions?	The AV node
What allows for rapid conduction of the action potential?	Bundle of HIS Bundle branch Purkinje fibers Specialized tracts
What is the sequence of the electrical impulse in the heart?	SA node → specialized tracts → AV node and atrial muscle → Bundle of HIS → bundle branches → Purkinje fibers → ventricle muscle

What serves to depress the heart rate at rest by slowing down the SA node?	Parasympathetic nervous system
How does the sympathetic nervous system affect conduction through the electrical system?	It speeds up conduction of the Action potential and therefore increases heart rate
What nerve has greatest influence on the heart?	The vagus nerve
What is the affect of vagal stimulation on the heart?	It serves to slow the conduction of action potentials through the AV node due to the parasympathetic nerve fibers it carries
How does norepi affect heart contractility?	It increases it
In which phase do the ventricles fill?	Late diastole
In which phase do we get isovolumic contraction?	Early systole
What phase of the cardiac cycle uses up most energy?	The isovolumic contraction of early systole
What is the purpose of isovolumic contraction?	To build up the pressure so as to overcome the high aortic pressure
In which phase is ejection?	In late systole
When is the relaxation phase?	Early diastole
What causes heart sound 1?	The closing of the atrial-ventricular valves
What causes heart sound 2?	The closing of the pulmonic and aortic valves
When in the cycle is heart sound 1?	Late diastole/early systole
When in the cycle is heart sound 2?	End systole begin diastole
What device records electrical activity of the heart?	Electrocardiograph
What information do we get from EKG?	Heart rate and rhythm Axis of the heart
What on an EKG marks atrial depolarization?	The P wave

What on an EKG marks ventricular depolarization?	The QRS complex
What on an EKG marks ventricular repolarization?	The T wave
What 2 things influence cardiac output?	Heart rate and stroke volume
What are the 3 major substrates for cardiac metabolism?	Fatty acids Glucose Glycogen breakdown
What are 3 minor substrates for cardiac metabolism?	Lactic acid Ketones Intramuscular triglycerides
What is the major limitation of energy metabolism by myocardium?	Coronary blood flow delivering oxygen
What 2 factors determine oxygen consumption by myocardium?	a. Wall tension in the heart that must be overcome e.g. during isovolumic contraction b. Isotonic contraction to eject the blood
What type of circulation has few controls, and is a low pressure/low resistance system?	The pulmonary system
What blood vessels act as capacitance vessels?	Veins and venules
What increases venous return?	Vasoconstriction
Which blood vessels have valves?	Veins and venules
What are the four pressures that affect capillary exchange?	a. Plasma oncotic pressure b. Plasma hydrostatic pressure c. Interstitial oncotic pressure d. Interstitial hydrostatic pressure
Which of the four pressures favors filtration?	a. Plasma hydrostatic pressure b. Interstitial oncotic pressure c. Interstitial hydrostatic pressure
Which of the four pressures is actually a negative pressure or "suction"?	Interstitial hydrostatic pressure

What are three mechanisms for edema?	a. Increased plasma interstitial pressure b. Decreased plasma oncotic pressure c. Increased interstitial oncotic pressure
How will decreased blood protein synthesis cause edema?	By decreasing plasma oncotic pressure.
What will influence lymph flow?	Smooth muscle tone Skeletal muscle contraction
Pressure in the right atrium or the vena cava at the level of the heart is known as what?	Central venous pressure
What will increase venous blood flow and decrease venous pressure?	Skeletal muscle contraction
Where are baroreceptors located?	In the aortic arch and carotids
What do baroreceptors sense?	Blood pressure changes
What cranial nerves innervate the baroreceptors?	Carotid sinus baroreceptor is innervated by CN IX Aortic arch baroreceptor is innervated by CN X
What kind (not type) of neurotransmitters are released when baroreceptors are stimulated by high blood pressure?	Inhibitory neurotransmitters
What do these inhibitory transmitters accomplish?	Inhibition of vasomotor and cardioregulatory centre of the medulla oblongata
How does the stimulation of the Cardioregulatory centre affect blood pressure?	Increased parasympathetic stimulation to the heart causes a decreased heart rate and contractile force
How does stimulationg the Vasomotor centre affet blood pressure?	Decreased sympathetic stimulation to blood vessels resulting in vasodilation
What is accomplished by stimulation baroreceptors?	A decrease in blood pressure due to the vasodilation
True or False: Baroreceptors can also increase blood pressure?	True, they can increase blood pressure along the same pathways
Where are chemoreceptors located?	Aortic arch and carotids

What are chemoreceptors sensitive to?	Low blood oxygen as a result of ↓ blood flow due to low blood pressure
What kind of neurotransmitter is released when chemoreceptors are stimulated by low pressure?	Excitatory neurotransmitters
What do these excitatory neurotransmitters do?	They increase the sympathetic firing down neurons that innervate smooth muscle of blood vessels which causes vasoconstriction
What is accomplished by stimulation of chemoreceptors?	An increase in blood pressure by vasoconstriction
How does increased vagal output cause decreased blood pressure?	Via its parasympathetic effects that cause a decreased heart rate leading to a decreased cardiac output leading to a decreased blood pressure
How does the kidney affect blood pressure?	Via renin angiotensin system: ↓ BP →↓ GFR → release of renin → eventually leads to release of aldosterone → kidneys reabsorb Na^+ and water →↑ Blood vol. →↑ BP
How does ADH affect BP?	Low BP →ADH release → kidney holds onto water →↑ blood vol. →↑ BP
In metabolic control of blood flow ↓ oxygen causes release of metabolites e.g. CO_2, lactate etc., which cause what?	Vasodilation of the blood vessels
What is the name of the control that protects against high pressure damage?	Autoregulation
What tissue is good at autoregulation?	Brain
What is the net result on blood vessels of autoregulation?	Vasoconstriction
What is the long term control of blood flow i.e. compensation for some type of tissue ischemia?	Angiogenesis
What is the primary catecholamine for alpha adrenergic receptors?	Norepinephrine

Which vascular beds have primarily alpha receptors?	Skin, renal and splanchnic vasculature
What affect does norepi have on smooth muscle cells in the vascular beds?	Vasoconstriction
What is the primary catecholamine for beta 2 receptors?	Epinephrine
Which vascular beds have primarily beta 2 receptors?	Coronary and skeletal muscle vessels
What affect does epi have on smooth muscle in the vascular beds?	Vasodilation
Which of the ANS branches has most control over circulation?	Sympathetics via Norepi and Epi (Vasoconstriction and vasodilation respectively)
Which vascular beds are overperfused at rest?	Skin, splanchnic and renal
Brain ischemia caused by an ↑ in CSF pressure is known as what?	Cushing's reflex
When, during the cardiac cycle, do the coronaries get their blood flow?	During diastole

Biochemistry

Which apolipoproteins (i.e. A, B, or C) are associated with which diseases?	Apo-A-V with hypertriglyceridemia Apo-B100 with hypobetalipoproteinemia Apo-C-II with hyperchylomicronemia Apo-C-III with hypertriglyceridemia
True or false: Cardiac muscle can use glucose, keton bodies, pyruvate, fatty acids, and lactate for fuel?	True, its preferred fuel is long-chain fatty acids with glucose as a second choice.
ATP is used in the heart for what?	60-70% of ATP is used for contraction and 40% is used for ion pumps
Why would hypophophatemia result in muscle weakness and impaired cardiac function?	Without a proper supply of both ADP and phosphate, then the Kreb Cycle cannot produce ATP

Besides raising LDL, triglycerides, and lipoprotein-a, what other affects do trans-fatty acids have on the cardiovascular system?	They promote inflammation, endothelial dysfunction, insulin resistance, visceral adiposity, and arrhythmias
Which minerals are associated with lowering blood pressure?	Magnesium, calcium, and potassium
B vitamin deficiency is associated with what cardiovascular disease?	cardiomyopathy
What polyphenol is associated with lowering blood pressure and has anti-oxidant, anti-platelet, and anti-inflammatory aproperties?	Flavonoids

Pathology

What are the two types of hemorrhage?	Acute— sudden, massive loss of blood Chronic— low-grade, mild leakage of blood
What are some of the complications of hemorrhage?	a. Hemorrhagic shock, which occurs when more than 15% of blood volume is lost. b. Hemorrhagic strokes, hemopericardium in areas sensitive to hemorrhage. c. Iron deficiency from chronic blood loss.
What is an exudate?	Edema fluid containing high amounts of protein and inflammatory cells
What is a transudate?	Edema fluid with a low protein content, not usually associated with inflammation
What mechanisms are involved in compensated, early, nonprogressive shock?	a. Increased heart rate and peripheral resistance to increase blood flow to vital organs b. Increased respiratory rate to remove carbon dioxide and raise pH
What occurs in the body during decompensated, progressive shock?	a. Oxygen levels fall, causing vasodilation and decreased blood flow to the heart b. Cell injury and cell death occurs from lack of oxygen

What occurs in the body during the irreversible stage of shock?	a. Acute tubular necrosis occurs in the kidney, which is initially reversible b. Full renal failure occurs as acute tubular necrosis becomes more severe c. Metabolic acidosis, coma and heart failure develop
What initiates clot (thrombus) formation?	Damage to endothelial cells that causes interactions between platelets, exposed collagen, and blood proteins.
What is the name of the factor that causes platelets to adhere to the exposed subendothelial surface in clot formation?	von Willebrand's factor
The extrinsic coagulation pathway is initiated by what tissue factor?	Thromboplastin
What causes thrombosis?	Abnormalities within the body that cause damage to endothelial cells, promote coagulation, or disturb blood flow.
What are the symptoms of chronic deep venous insufficiency in the legs?	Pigmentation, edema, skin induration, ulceration
What is the most common cause of death in Western industrialized countries?	Arterial thrombosis (atherosclerosis) due primarily to cigarette smoking
What is an embolus?	A piece of a thrombus that has broken off, entered the bloodstream, and become trapped in the vasculature (thromboembolism)
Where do leg venous thrombi commonly lodge?	In the lung, after entering the right atrium of the heart through the inferior vena cava and passing through the ventricle (pulmonary emboli)
Where do arterial emboli that break off from mural thrombi in the heart or major arteries commonly lodge?	a. Branches of the carotid artery, causing stroke b. Branches of the mesenteric artery, causing hemorrhagic infarction c. Branches of the renal artery, causing renal cortex infarcts

What is the name of an embolus that lodges at the bifurcation of the main pulmonary artery?	Saddle embolus
What are the two types of infarcts?	a. Anemic— white or pale in areas without collateral blood supply b. Hemorrhagic— red, in areas where collateral blood supply may be insufficient
What causes infarction?	Blockage or lack of blood flow to an organ
How is arteriosclerosis defined?	Sclerosis (hardening) of the arteries
What types of arteries are affected by atherosclerosis?	Atherosclerosis is arteriosclerosis of large elastic arteries, including the aorta, coronary, common iliac, femoral, popliteal, internal carotid, and cerebral arteries
What are atheromas?	Lesions that develop on artery walls comprised of macrophages, low-density lipoproteins (LDL), fibrin, and smooth muscle. They are usually asymptomatic for 20–40 years until they become symptomatic, complicated plaques
How does arteriosclerosis most probably begin?	Damage to vascular endothelium
When oxidized lipids are ingested by macrophages, what do they form?	Foam cells
What stages are involved in polyarteritis nodosa (PAN)?	a. Immune complex deposits in walls of arteries in the first stage, initiating the complement cascade and calling in neutrophils b. Macrophages and fibroblasts replace neutrophils in the healing stage, and fibrosis occurs c. In the last stage, a cord of collagen forms in the vessel with calcium deposits, occluding the lumen
What is a hallmark of PAN?	To find lesions in all three stages of development in one vessel

What is the most common form of vasculitis?	Temporal arteritis
What does thromboangitis obliterans (Buerger's disease) cause?	Ischemia, pain, gangrene, necrosis of the digits
How is Raynaud's phenomenon different from Raynaud's disease?	Raynaud's phenomenon is usually secondary to an underlying disorder, such as scleroderma or lupus, while Raynaud's disease occurs independently.
Where do aneurysms occur?	Arteries that are weak or thin
What are two common types of aneurysms?	a. Atherosclerotic aneurysms—occur in abdominal aorta or iliac arteries b. Berry aneurysms—congenital defects in cerebral arteries, most usually the Circle of Willis
How does the heart adapt to hypertension?	a. Increase wall thickness → cardiac hypertrophy b. To dilate the heart chamber (Frank starling mechanism)→ Cardiac dilation
What occurs in an aortic dissection?	The aortic intima tears, allowing blood to enter other histologic layers, and potentially leading to aortic rupture
What is the most dangerous form of varicose veins?	Esophageal varices
What are the two versions of venous thrombosis?	a. Acute inflammation of the vein (thrombophlebitis) b. No inflammation (phlebothrombosis)
What conditions promote thrombosis?	Blood stasis in the legs from immobilization, cardiac failure, pregnancy or varicose veins.
What are common hemangiomas?	Port wine stains, strawberry marks, cavernous hemangiomas, and vascular spiders
When the heart experiences chronic or acute insults, what happens first?	Compensation

What occurs with right-sided congestive heart failure (CHF)?	a. Imbalance in Frank-Starling forces b. Leading to dilation c. Hypertrophy and enlargement d. Failure of the right ventricle
What causes right-sided congestive heart failure?	Secondary to left-sided CHF or lung disease (cor pulmonale)
What occurs with left-sided congestive heart failure?	a. Imbalance in Frank-Starling forces b. Dilation c. Hypertrophy and enlargement d. Failure of the left ventricle
What causes left-sided congestive heart failure?	Acute myocardial infarction
What mechanisms of compensation are involved in congestive heart failure?	a. Baroreceptor response b. Shift in oxygen-hemoglobin dissociation curve c. Increase in blood volume d. Myocyte hypertrophy
What four basic syndromes occur with ischemic heart disease?	Angina pectoris Myocardial infarction Chronic ischemic heart disease Sudden cardiac death
What causes ischemic heart disease?	Reduced coronary blood flow, increased myocardial demand, and decreased oxygen in the blood
What are the two types of damage that occur with myocardial infarction (MI)?	a. Transmural— entire cardiac wall develops myocardial necrosis b. Subendocardial— inner one-third of heart wall develops myocardial necrosis
What is the most common form of angina?	Stable angina
Which forms of angina are helped by nitroglycerin?	Stable angina and Prinzmetal's angina
Which form of angina is not helped by nitroglycerin?	Unstable angina

What are some of the complications of ischemic heart disease after MI?	Arrhythmias Myocardial rupture Mural thrombosis and embolism Ventricular aneurysm Ruptured papillary muscle
What is rheumatic heart disease?	Negative sequelae from infection with Group A beta hemolytic Streptococcus pyogenes
How does rheumatic heart disease develop?	A Type II hypersensitivity reaction causes a cross-reaction of strep antibodies with heart tissue. Inflammation of all layers of the heart and damage to heart valves occurs
What physical signs are associated with mitral valve prolapse?	a. Audible midsystolic click b. A late systolic murmur consistent with mitral regurgitation
Where is an aortic stenosis murmur best heard?	Apex, though it may radiate to the carotids
What causes acute endocarditis?	Staphylococcus aureus, secondary to systemic infection
What causes subacute bacterial endocarditis?	Less virulent organisms, such as Streptococcus viridans
What are some common causes of myocardial infections?	a. Bacterial, such as staph, strep and diphtheria b. Rickettsial, such as typhus, Rocky Mountain Spotted Fever c. Viral, including Coxsackie, influenza and echo viruses d. Parasitic, including toxoplasmosis, trichinosis
What is dilated cardiomyopathy?	Cardiomyopathy leading to ventricular dilation, commonly caused by the death of myocardial cells.
What is restrictive cardiomyopathy?	Cardiomyopathy with rigid ventricular walls, the most rare type.

What is hypertrophic cardiomyopathy?	Congenital, acquired or idiopathic cardiomyopathy with significant ventricular hypertrophy.
As of 2009, hypertrophic cardiomyopathy, dilated cardiomyopathy, and arrhythmogenic right ventricular dysplasia have been linked with what causative factor?	A mutation of a single gene that results in altered structural proteins.
Hemopericardium may cause what condition?	Cardiac tamponade, a restriction in the filling of the heart.
What are the three types of acute pericarditis?	a. Fibrinous—caused by uremia, viral infection, myocardial infarction b. Purulent—caused by bacterial infection c. Hemorrhagic
Chronic fibrosing pericarditis may cause what condition?	Constrictive pericarditis
Serous pericarditis is also known by what other name?	Pericardial effusion
What four congenital defects are found in tetralogy of Fallot?	Ventricular septal defect Pulmonary stenosis Overriding aorta Hypertrophy of the right ventricle
What are the most common congenital heart defects?	Interventricular septal defects
What are some of the causes of chronic cor pulmonale?	COPD Pulmonary interstitial fibrosis Cystic fibrosis Pulmonary arteritis Chest movement disorders Metabolic acidosis

Endrocrine System

Embryology

What tissue invaginates to form the anterior lobe of the pituitary gland?	Ectodermal tissue of the oropharynx
This invagination is known as what?	The Rathke's pouch, which eventually extends downward to the hypothalamus and becomes the pituitary stalk
From what does the posterior lobe of the pituitary gland arise?	The neural crest
What does the pancreas form from?	From two diverticular buds of the foregut
By what week have the first islets of the pancreas appeared?	Around week 10, they first appear in the tail of the pancreas.
From what tissue does the thyroid develop?	It starts developing in the primitive ailmentary tract and consists of endodermal cells
Where does the thyroid first develop?	In the buccal cavity
What structure does the thyroid gland help to develop as it matures?	The tongue
What is embryonic connection do the tongue and thyroid share?	The thyroglossal duct
Where on the tongue does the thyroglossal duct open?	The foramen cecum

From which pouches do the parathyroid glands develop?	The superior gland decends from the fourth pharyngeal pouch and the inferior glands from the third pharyngeal pouch
True or false: The adrenal cortex and medulla develop from the same embryonic line	False, the cortex develops from coelomic mesodermal tissue and the medulla arises from ectodermal tissue of the neural crest
Between the adrenal cortex and the medulla, which develops parallel with the sympathetic nervous system?	The adrenal medulla

Anatomy

What sits in the hypophoseal fossa of the sella turcica of the sphenoid bones?	Pituitary gland
What is located posterior to the thalamus and superior to the midbrain of the brainstem?	Pineal gland
What is the body's largest endocrine gland?	Thyroid
Describe the location of the thyroid by bony landmarks	Located between levels of C_5 and T_1 vertebrae, on the anterior aspect of the neck below the cricoid cartilage
How many parathyroid glands do you usually have?	4
Where are the superior and inferior parathyroid glands located?	The superior glands are on the thyroid's posteromedial aspect near the tracheoesophageal groove The inferior parathyroids are located below the inferior thyroid artery
What are the 2 parts of the adrenal gland?	Cortex Medulla
Superior to what organ would you find each adrenal gland?	Kidney
What are the 3 layers of the adrenal cortex?	Glomerulosa Fasciculata Reticularis

What does each layer secrete?	Glomerulosa secrets mineralcorticoids (e.g. aldosterone) Fasciculata secretes glucocorticoids (e.g. cortisol) Reticularis secrets androgrens (e.g. Dehydropiandrosterone)
What cells produce catecholamines in the adrenal glands?	Chromaffin cells

Physiology

What do we call a chemical substance released by an endocrine gland into the blood in which it travels to another site in the body where it exerts its effect?	A hormone
What are the 3 classes of hormones?	a. Derived from amino acids b. Protein or peptide based c. Steroids
What amino acid serves as the starting point of most of the amino acid derived hormones?	Tyrosine
What 2 organs release tyrosine based hormones?	a. Thyroid gland → thyroxine b. Adrenal medulla → Epi and Norepi
What type of receptor when bound to hormone causes an increase in cAMP?	Plasmalemma receptors
cAMP is an example of what?	Second messenger
What is the effect of an ↑ in cAMP?	It causes an ↑ in cytosolic calcium
What substances use plasmalemma receptors?	Polypeptide hormones like Norepi and Epi
What receptors use cytoplasmic receptors?	Steroids
How do steroids interact with the cytoplasmic receptor?	They bind to the receptor and the whole complex binds to DNA and induces gene expression to produce new proteins
What substances use nuclear receptors?	T3 and T4

What is the effect of T3 binding to a nuclear receptor?	↑ transcription and ↑ translation (production of proteins)
GH, ACTH, TSH, FSH, LH, and prolactin come from where?	Anterior pituitary
How is the hypothalmus and anterior pituitary connected?	Via portal vessels
What gland is controlled by hypothalamic releasing substances?	Anterior pituitary (adenohypophysis)
What gland is controlled by nerve signals from the hypothalmus?	Posterior pituitary (neurohypophysis)
What stimulates growth of ovum and sperm?	FSH
What stimulates the maturation and release of ovum?	LH
What stimulates the liver to release somatomedians?	Growth hormone
What promotes protein synthesis and uptake of various amino acids?	Growth hormone
What promotes ↑ use of fats, release of fatty acids, ↓ use of carbohydrates and ↑ beta oxidation?	Growth hormone
Where are ADH and oxytocin released from?	Posterior pituitary
What stimulates the release of GH from the Anterior pituitary?	GHRH
What stimulates the release of GHRH from the hypothalmus?	Stress: malnutrition (especially protein), hypoglycemia, exercise, physical/mental trauma
How does hypothalamus affect posterior pituitary?	Hormones are produced by hypothalmus and are transported down nerve endings to the posterior pituitary
What is target tissue for ADH?	Kidney collecting ducts

What is main stimulus for release of ADH?	↑ blood osmolarity sensed by hypothalmus
What mineral is important for synthesis of thyroid hormones?	Iodine
What is the active form of thyroid hormone?	T3/triiodothyroxine
In what form is most of the thyroid hormone in the body?	T4/thyroxine
How is thyroxin transported in blood?	It is bound to thyroxin binding globulin, prealbumin, or albumin
What stimulates release of TRH?	Cold, emotional reactions, ↑ calories
What is the function of thyroid hormone?	To maintain basal metabolic rate
How does thyroid hormone maintain basal metabolic rate?	By ↑ activity of Na^+/K^+ ATPase pump
What is the effect of calcitonin on the body?	Decreases blood calcium levels
How does calcitonin decrease blood calcium?	↓ activity of Ca^{2+} pump ↑ osteoblastic activity → bone formation ↓ osteoclastic activity → less bone turnover
Where is calcitonin released?	Thyroid gland, C cells
What does parathyroid hormone do?	↑ calcium levels in the blood
How does PTH ↑ calcium levels in the blood?	↑ intestinal absorption of calcium (with Vit. D3) ↑ kidney reabsorption ↑ bone resorption
What are the two major controls of blood calcium?	PTH Vitamin D3
Where are catecholamines produced?	Adrenal medulla
The adrenal medulla functions most like what kind of neuron?	Post ganglionic sympathetic neuron

What four classes of hormones are released from adrenal cortex?	a. Glucocoticoids b. Mineralcorticoids c. Androgens d. Estrogens and progesterones
How is cortisol transported?	Bound to globulins Bound to albumin Free form
The fact that we need cortisol in small levels for other hormones to work is known as what?	Permissive effect
What stimulates cortisol release?	ACTH
ACTH exhibits diurnal variations. When is it at its highest?	In the morning
What else is produced along with ACTH?	MSH- melanocyte stimulating hormone
What are some of the anabolic physiological activities of cortisol?	a. Stimulates gluconeogenesis b. Stimulates glycogen breakdown c. Stimulates protein synthesis
What are some of the catabolic effects of cortisol at physiological doses?	1. ↑ Protein catabolism in skeletal muscle, connective tissue, and lymphoid tissue 2. ↑ Lipolysis 3. ↑ Production of rate-limiting enzymes for gluconeogenesis
What are some of the other roles of cortisol at physiological doses?	Weak aldosterone effect Stimulates surfactant production in fetuses Anti inflammatory Enhances immune function
What stimulates CRF?	Stress e.g. hypoglycemia, intense hot or cold, chronic pain, emotions, disease
What is the major mineralcorticoid?	Aldosterone
What are the target tissues for aldosterone?	Kidney Sweat glands Salivary glands Colonic epithelium

What are the major effects of aldosterone?	Regulation of blood volume and blood pressure
How does aldosterone regulate blood volume and pressure?	a. By causing an ↑ in Na^+ reabsorption → ↑ water reabsorption b. ↑ K^+ excretion
What is the long term control of aldosterone?	Angiotensin II
What are some of the other controls of aldosterone?	↑ K^+ (potent regulator) ↓ Na^+
What is needed for aldosterone to work?	ACTH
What is the major adrenal androgen?	DHEA
What hormone promotes fuel storage?	Insulin
What will increase insulin release?	High blood glucose Sweet tasting food Amino acids
What hormones increase insulin levels?	GI hormones →CCK, secretin and gastrin Cortisol
What inhibits insulin release?	Epi and norepi and somatostatin
What are the effects of insulin?	↑ Cellular uptake of glucose ↑ Glucose utilization ↑ Glycogen synthesis ↑ Fatty acid synthesis ↑ Protein synthesis
What hormone is released with low blood sugar?	Glucagon
What are the main stimuli for release of glucagon?	Main stimuli →↓ blood sugar ↑ Blood amino acids Epi/Norepi
What are some of the effects of glucagon?	↑ Blood glucose via: ↑ Gluconeogenesis ↑ Glycogenolysis ↑ Triglyceride breakdown in adipose tissue

Biochemistry

What kind of hormones act on plasma membrane receptors coupled with regulatory molecules like G proteins?	Water-soluble hormones (ex: amino-acid based hormones, except the thyroid hormone)
What kind of hormones act on intracellular receptors?	Lipid-soluble hormones (ex. steriod hormones)
What are some example of second messengers?	DAG and IP3
Which hormone has the greatest control over free fatty acid release from adipose tissue?	Catecholamines. They bind to beta-adrenergic receptors and activate G protein activity.
Which other hormones activate lipolysis in adipose tissue?	Glucagon, adrenocorticotropic hormone, alpha-melanocyte-stimulating hormone, and thyroid-stimulating hormone.
What hormones are needed to stimulate conversion of cholesterol to pregnenolone in endocrine organs?	Adrenocorticotropin hormone in the adrenals and luteinizing hormone in the ovaries and testes
The process by which androgens are transformed into estrogens is called what?	Aromatization, because the reactions are catalyzed by the aromatase enzyme.
What steroid hormones can peripheral or non-endocrine tissue create?	Adipose tissue can, using aromatase enzymes, convert androsternedione to estrones The Skin can convert testosterone into dihydrotestosterone (DHT)
Which hormones secreted by the anterior pituitary are protein-based?	Growth hormone, thyroid-stimulating hormone, adrenocorticotropin hormone, follicle stimulating hormone, luteinizing hormone, and prolactin releasing hormone
What stimulates IGFS?	Growth Hormone
What effect does (IGFS) have in the body?	Stimulates amino acid uptake and movement from the blood to cells Stimulates cell growth and proliferation Stimulates uptake of sulfur into cartilage matrix Increases skeletal growth

| What common beverage inhibits ADH release? | Alcohol, thus it results in copious urine output |

Pathology

| What hormones are secreted by the most common adenomas, causing hyperpituitarism? | a. Prolactinomas— secrete prolactin
b. Somatotrope adenomas— secrete growth hormone
c. Corticotrope adenomas— secrete ACTH
d. Gonadotrope adenomas— secrete FSH and LH
e. Thyrotrope adenomas— secrete TSH |

| What are some of the causes of hypopituitarism? | a. Adenoma impinging on pituitary
b. Loss of blood supply
c. Congenital agenesis
d. Metastatic cancer |

| What occurs with diabetes insipidus? | Decreased ADH causes polydipsia and polyuria |

| An open embryonic thyroglossal duct can cause what? | Thyroglossal duct cysts and fistulas with the potential for infection or in papillary cancer |

| What are the symptoms of Graves' disease? | a. Diffuse toxic goiter
b. Nervousness
c. Palpitations
d. Rapid pulse
e. Fatigability
f. Weight loss
g. Sweating
h. Emotional lability
i. Menstrual changes
j. Exophthalmos |

| How does cretinism present in newborns? | Apathy
Sluggishness
Severe mental retardation
Stunted growth
Low body temperature |

Hashimoto's thyroiditis is associated with what autoimmune conditions?	a. Systemic lupus erythematosus (SLE) b. Rheumatoid arthritis c. Graves' disease d. Pernicious anemia e. Sjogren's syndrome
What are the phases of subacute thyroiditis?	Phase one: thryotoxicosis Phase two: hypothyroidism Phase three: recovery to euthyroid state
Granulomatous and silent subacute thyroiditis are most often seen after what type of infection?	Viral infection
What are some causes of goiters?	a. Physiologic enlargement b. Iodine deficiency c. Hashimoto's thyroiditis d. Goitrogens e. Failure of thyroid hormone synthesis
What are hot nodules?	Thyroid adenomas are benign nodules that are highly active and take up radioactive iodine
What are the characteristics of thyroid cancer?	They are slow growing nodules that have lost function and do not take up radioactive iodine
Medullary carcinoma of the thyroid (MTC) is genetically associated with what conditions?	Multiple endocrine neoplasia types 2A and 2B
When is parathyroid hormone normally secreted?	It is secreted in response to low blood calcium levels. It increases reabsorption of calcium
What causes primary hyperparathyroidism?	Parathyroid adenoma
What causes secondary hyperparathyroidism?	Decreased serum calcium as a result of chronic renal disease
What three types of hormones are produced by the adrenal cortex?	a. Mineralocorticoids— aldosterone b. Glucocorticoids— cortisol c. Androgens— DHEA

What is aldosterone's effect in the body?	It increases sodium and water reabsorption by the kidneys
What are the symptoms of Cushing's syndrome?	a. Redistribution of body fat b. Skin atrophy with easy bruising and striae c. Hirsutism d. Muscle weakness e. Osteoporosis f. Amenorrhea g. Hypertension h. Hyperglycemia i. Psychiatric dysfunction
What is Conn's syndrome?	Primary aldosteronism usually due to adrenocortical adenoma or hyperplasia that causes hyperproduction of adrenal mineralocorticoids.
What is Addison's disease?	Adrenal gland fails to produce cortisol, aldosterone, and androgens, causing hypotension, increased pigmentation of the skin, increased serum potassium, decreased serum sodium, chloride, glucose and bicarbonate.
What is produced in the adrenal medulla?	Epinephrine and norepinephrine
What is the primary symptom of pheochromocytoma?	Paroxysmal or persistent hypertension
Where is insulin produced?	Pancreatic islet beta cells
Where is glucagon produced?	Alpha cells of the pancreas
What causes type I diabetes mellitus?	Failure of the beta cells of the pancreas to produce insulin from either autoimmune or genetic causes
What causes type II diabetes mellitus?	Increased insulin resistance of cells associated with central obesity and sedentary lifestyle

How do insulinomas clinically present?

Increased insulin secretion, confusion, anxiety, stupor, convulsions, and coma (Whipple's triad)

What is the Zollinger-Ellison syndrome?

A gastroduodenal hyperacidity syndrome caused by a gastrin-secreting tumor (gastrinoma) in the pancreas or intestinal wall

Gastrointestinal System

Embryology

What germ layer forms the excretory organs?	Mesoderm
What germ layer forms the glands opening into the GI tract?	Endoderm
What germ layer forms the glandular cells of the liver and pancreas?	Endoderm
What germ layer forms the lining of the GI tract?	Endoderm
What remnant persists after the joining of the embryonic palantine processes and is located on the soft palate?	The palantine raphe
The embryonic ductus venosus becomes what after birth?	Ligamentum venosum
The embryonic umbilical vein becomes what after birth?	Ligamentum teres
The embryonic umbilical arteries become what after birth?	Umbilical ligament

Anatomy

To which bones are the teeth attached?	The superior teeth attaches to the maxilla the inferior teeth attach to the mandible
How many permanent teeth are there?	32
How many deciduous teeth are there?	20
What nerve supplies the teeth?	The superior and inferior alveolar nerves
What glandular duct opens at level of 2nd maxillary molars?	Parotid gland
What innervates touch and taste for the epiglottis?	CN X (vagus)
What nerve innervates the upper 1/3 of the striate muscle of the esophagus?	Vagus (CN X)
Where does peristalsis occur in the esophagus?	Inferior 2/3
What passes through the diaphragm?	The esophagus The aorta Inferior vena cava
At what spinal level are the aortic opening, esophageal opening, and the caval opening (i.e. where the inferior vena cava and the right phrenic nerve pass through) in the diaphragm?	Aortic opening at T12 The esophageal opening at T10 The caval opening at T8
True or False: The diaphragm, external and internal intercostals and transverse thoracic muscle are all innervated by the intercostal nerves.	False, the diaphragm is innervated by the phrenic nerve and the other 3 are innervated by the intercostal nerves.
What organs are retroperitoneal?	Duodenum Ascending and descending colon Kidney Pancreas (at least part of it)
What are the 4 lobes of the liver?	Right Left Quadrate Caudate

What tunnels through liver to collect filtered blood?	Inferior vena cava
What does the hepatic triad consist of?	Hepatic artery Hepatic vein Bile duct
Where does the liver tissue get its blood from?	Hepatic artery from the celiac trunk
What separates the right from the left lobe of the liver?	Falciform ligament
What attaches the liver to the abdominal wall?	Round ligament
What is the name of the transverse fissure where ducts and vessels enter and leave the liver on the visceral surface between the caudate and quadrate lobes?	Porta hepatis
What are the 2 sources of blood for the liver?	Hepatic artery Portal vein
What separates the quadrate lobe of the liver from the left lobe on visceral surface?	Ligamentum teres
Describe the musculature of the stomach from inside out.	Internal-oblique Middle-circular Outer-longitudinal
What artery supplies the stomach?	The celiac via the L and R gastric arteries
The greater curvature of the stomach is suplied by which arteries?	R and L gastroepiploic arteries
The lesser curvature of the stomach is supplied by which arteries?	R and L gastric arteries
What are the 3 branches of the celiac trunk?	Left gastric Common hepatic Splenic
What organs receive blood from the celiac trunk?	Stomach Liver Spleen

What are the 3 main veins that drain into the portal vein?	Splenic Superior mesenteric Inferior mesenteric
What kind of nerves are splanchnic nerves?	Sympathetics
What action do the splanchnic nerves have on the stomach?	↓ peristalsis and acid secretion
What provides the parasympathetics to the stomach?	Vagus nerve (CN X)
What action do parasympathetics have on the stomach?	↑ peristalsis and acid secretion
What vein drains the stomach?	The gastric vein, which drains into the portal vein
How do pancreatic enzymes enter duodenum?	Through the duodenal papilla
Which part of the S.I. does most absorption?	Jejunum
Which part of the S.I. has larger diameter, larger villi and longer vasa recta (straight arteries)?	Jejunum
Which part of the S.I. has more arterial arcades and more peyers patches?	Ileum
In which part of the S.I. is vitamin B12 absorbed?	Terminal ileum
What artery supplies blood to the S.I.?	Superior mesenteric artery
What vein drains the S.I.?	Superior mesenteric vein
Where does the lacteal transport fat?	To the thoracic duct
What are the thickened bands of longitudinal smooth muscle of the L.I. called?	Teniae coli
What are the pouches of the colon called?	Haustra
Which parts of the colon are retroperitoneal?	Ascending and descending portions

What vascular beds in the anus can cause internal hemorrhages?	Rectal venous plexus
What nerve innervates the skeletal muscle of the external anal sphincter?	Pudendal nerve
What parts of the large intestine does the superior mesenteric supply?	Ileocecal area Ascending colon 1/2 of transverse colon
What parts of the L.I. does the inferior mesenteric artery supply?	1/2 of transverse colon Descending colon Sigmoid Rectum
Where are three areas of concern for varicosities caused by hypertension?	Esophagus - bleeding varicies Anal canal - hemorrhoids Umbilicus
Where do the parasympathetics that supply the L.I. come from?	S 2,3,4, pelvic splanchnics

Physiology

What are the 2 types of tissue that forms the spleen?	Red pulp White pulp
What are the 2 motor activities of the mouth?	Mastication Deglutition (swallowing)
What is the motor activity of the esophagus? How is this accomplished?	Propulsion by peristalsis
What are the 3 motor activities of the stomach?	Mixing Storage Emptying
What 2 things regulate stomach emptying?	Gastrin Stomach distention
How do long chain fatty acids affect stomach emptying?	They decrease it by causing release of CCK which inhibits gastrin
How does duodenal distention and irritation affect stomach emptying time?	The decrease emptying time

What is the purpose of rhythmic segmentation in the S.I.?	To mix up the chyme to expose it to enzymes and absorptive surface
What structure prevents backflow from colon and separates S.I. bugs from L.I. bugs?	Ileocecal valve/sphincter
What causes the sphincter to relax?	Gastric distention via gastroileal reflex Gastrin
Where does most of the water absorption take place?	In cecum and transverse colon
What does rectal dissension cause?	A desire to defecate
What are the 2 types of electrical activity in the G.I.?	Slow waves (Basic Electrical Rhythm BER) Spike potentials
Which of the 2 types of electrical activity leads to smooth muscle contraction?	Spike potentials
Which of the 2 electrical activities keeps G.I. in a state of readiness by helping set up gut tone?	Slow waves
What helps set up frequency and rhythm of action potential and smooth muscle contraction?	Slow waves
Which branch of the ANS has most affect on the G.I.?	Parasympathetics
What are the 2 areas of intrinsic nervous control on the gut?	Myenteric (Auerbach's) plexus Submucosal (Meissner's) plexus
Which of the 2 plexuses controls motility and contraction?	Myenteric plexus
Which of the 2 plexuses controls secretions?	Submucosal plexus
Which of the 2 extrinsic nervous system controls will ↓ blood flow leading to decreased secretions?	Sympathetics
Which of the 2 extrinsic nervous system controls will ↑ motility and secretions?	Parasympathetics

What are the antibacterial substances found in saliva?	Lactoferrin- binds iron to prevent bacterial cell growth IgA Muramidase (Breaks down bacterial cell walls)
What enzymes are found in saliva?	Lingual lipase Amylase
What affect does ↑ parasympathetics have on saliva secretion?	It will ↑ rate of secretion
What are some of the functions of HCL?	a. Activation of pepsinogen into pepsin b. Provides the adequate pH for pepsin activity, micronutrient absorption c. Storage and mixing up of chyme d. Denatures proteins e. Antibacterial
What is secreted from parietal cells?	HCL Intrinsic factor
What is secreted from chief cells?	Pepsinogen
What is secreted from goblet cells?	Mucous
What breaks down the aromatic amino acid bonds of proteins?	Pepsin
What are 3 stimulants for HCL secretion?	a. Parasympathetics b. Gastrin release stimulated by stomach distention and secretagogues c. Histamine
What neutralizes the acidic chyme as it moves into the duodenum?	Bicarbonate
What causes release of bicarbonate?	Secretin
Where are zymogen granules produced and released from? (organ and cells)	From acinar cells in pancreas
Which pancreatic cells secrete both insulin and glucagon?	Islet of Langerhans or Pancreatic islets
Which cells produce bicarbonate?	Ductal cells

What activates trypsinogen into trypsin?	Enterokinase
What activates the remaining zymogens?	Trypsin
What is major stimulus for zymogen release?	CCK
What stimulates release of CCK?	Fat in S.I. Partially digested proteins
What hormone enhances activity of CCK?	Insulin
What 2 hormones inhibit pancreatic juice production and activity?	Somatostatin Glucagon
What action does acetylcholine have on pancreatic secretions?	It will ↑ secretion due to parasympathetic action
What does gelatinase breakdown?	Proteoglycans that are present in connective tissue of flesh products
Facilitated diffusion of sugars across gut epithelium is dependent on Co-transport of what?	Sodium
What does the P450 system do to xenobiotics?	Makes them more hydrophilic with addition of -OH group
What are the active phagocytes of the liver?	Kupffer cells

Biochemistry

Basic Carbohydrate Biochemistry

What 2 monosaccharides make up lactose?	Galactose and glucose
What 2 monosaccharides make up sucrose?	Glucose and fructose
Which polysaccharide is composed of glucose units linked by alpha-1,4 linkages?	Amylose
What polysaccharide has glucose linked by alpha-1,4 and alpha-1,6 linkages?	Glycogen
What polysaccharide has long chains of alpha-1,4 linkages and every 25 molecules has an alpha-1,6 branch?	Amylopectin

What polysaccharide has glucose molecules bound at beta 1,4 linkages?	Cellulose
Which disaccharide has 2 glucose units?	Maltose
Salivary and pancreatic amylase breaks down what type of linkages?	Alpha-1,4
Maltase cleaves which linkage?	Alpha-1,4
Isomaltase cleaves which linkage?	Alpha-1,6
The enzymes maltase, sucrase, dextrinase and lactase are found where?	In the brush borders of the mucosal cells
What is the rate limiting enzyme in the reaction of fructose to glucose?	Fructokinase
What is the rate limiting enzyme in the reaction of galactose to glucose?	Galactokinase
Dextrin is only released from the hydrolysis of which polysaccharide?	Amylopectin
What hormone is released when glucose levels are high?	Insulin
Which organ keeps a constant level of glucose in the blood by storing and producing it as needed?	The liver
Which tissues do not require insulin to take up glucose?	The liver, brain, RBC
Which hormones are released when glucose levels are down?	Glucagon, epinephrine, cortisol
Which of the catecholamines stimulates gluconeogenesis?	Epinephrine
Glucokinase is only found in which organ?	The liver
In what part of the cell does glycolysis occur?	Cytosol of the cytoplasm

What enzyme allows the liver to trap glucose in the form of glucose-6-phosphate?	Glucokinase
What are the 3 rate-limiting enzymes of glycolysis?	Hexokinase/glucokinase Phosphofructokinase Pyruvate kinase
How many molecules of pyruvate do we get from one molecule of glucose?	2
What mineral is required for the phosphorylation reactions of glucokinase and phosphofructokinase?	Magnesium
What is the net harvest from aerobic glycolysis?	8 ATP (2 ATP, +6 ATP from 2 NADH, +4 ATP)
Which Krebs cycle intermediate inhibits action of phosphofructokinase and therefore inhibits glycolysis?	Citrate
What is the net harvest of anaerobic glycolysis?	2 ATP (NADH still gets produced but under anaerobic conditions does not get oxidized)
What is the aerobic fate of pyruvate?	Acetyl-CoA
Under anaerobic conditions pyruvate is reduced to what?	Lactate
What enzyme complex converts pyruvate into Acetyl-CoA?	Pyruvate dehydrogenase complex
What vitamins are needed for the pyruvate dehydrogenase complex?	Vitamin B1 or thiamin Vitamin B2 in the form of FAD Vitamin B3 in the form of NAD Vitamin B5 in the form of CoA
What mineral is required for the pyruvate dehydrogenase complex?	Magnesium
Pyruvate carboxylase converts pyruvate into what?	Oxaloacetate
What cofactor is important in the carboxylation reaction of pyruvate to oxaloacetate?	Biotin

Why is the production of oxaloacetate from pyruvate important?	In order for the Krebs cycle to run
What acts to promote pyruvate dehydrogenase and the subsequent formation of Acetyl-CoA?	The presence of pyruvate
What inhibits pyruvate dehydrogenase and promotes pyruvate carboxylase thus shuttling pyruvate into oxaloacetate?	The presence of Acetyl-CoA
Where does the Krebs cycle take place?	In the mitochondria
In which cells does the Krebs cycle not take place?	RBC, as they lack mitochondria
Which metabolite of the Krebs cycle is used for fatty acid synthesis?	Citrate
Which 2 Krebs cycle metabolites are important for amino acid synthesis?	Oxaloacetate and alpha ketoglutarate
Which Krebs cycle metabolite is used in porphyrin/heme metabolism?	Succinyl-CoA
Acetyl-CoA joins with what substance to form citrate?	Oxaloacetate
What regulates the Krebs cycle?	The ratio of ADP to ATP
What does high levels of ATP do to the Krebs cycle?	It slows it down
What coenzymes are needed in the Krebs cycle?	B3 as NAD B2 as FAD B5 to make Succinyl-CoA
Name four uses for Acetyl-CoA.	1. ATP production 2. Fatty acid synthesis 3. Ketone synthesis 4. Cholesterol formation
Which enzyme regulates the levels of Acetyl-CoA?	Pyruvate dehydrogenase complex
What are the 2 reducing equivalents?	NAD and FAD

What metabolite of the Krebs cycle is an important indicator of energy status of the cell?	Citrate
How is oxaloacetate transported out of the mitochondrion?	Via conversion to malate
In what organs does gluconeogenesis occur?	Mostly liver but also kidney
Which hormone by its involvement with glucagon inhibits glycolysis and promotes gluconeogenesis?	Epinephrine
What steroid hormone promotes the gluconeogenic pathway?	Cortisol
Name 3 substrates for gluconeogenesis.	1. Alanine (and other amino acids) 2. Glycerol 3. Lactate
What are the 2 key products of the hexose monophosphate shunt?	NADPH Ribose (used in nucleotide synthesis)
What is the harvest from the Krebs cycle?	3 NADH 1 FADH 1 GTP
What is the key rate-limiting enzyme in glycogen synthesis?	Glycogen synthase
What hormone activates glycogen synthase?	Insulin
What hormones inhibit glycogen synthesis?	Cortisol, glucagon
What substance in low quantities inhibits glycogen synthase?	cAMP
Which tissues have high amounts of glycogen?	Liver and skeletal muscle
Which metabolite in glycolysis is transformed into glycogen?	Glucose-6-phosphate
What substance carries glucose molecules to the growing glycogen chain?	UDP

What is the rate-limiting enzyme in glycogenolysis?	Phosphorylase
How is NADPH used by the body?	It maintains iron as Fe2+ in RBCs
How many ATP do you get from NADH?	3
How many ATP from FADH?	2
Where does FADH enter the electron transport chain?	At ubiquinone
What mineral is important in the electron transport chain?	Iron
What is the overall harvest of energy from 1 molecule of glucose?	8 ATP from glycolysis 2 NADH from pyruvate to acetyl SCoA →6 ATP 6 NADH→18 ATP 2 FADH→4 ATP 2 GTP→2 ATP Total of 38 ATP
What is the final electron acceptor in the electron transport chain?	Oxygen
The process of forming ATP from electrons is called what?	Transduction

Basic Lipid Biochemistry

What is the action of lipase?	It breaks down ester bonds
What is the optimal pH for gastric lipases?	4.5 to 6.0
Where does lipolysis of dietary triglycerides occur?	20–30% in the stomach, 80–70% in the small intestines
What constitutes a triglyceride?	3 Fatty acids attached to a glycerol backbone
Lecithin or phosphotadylcholine is found in what substance?	Phospholipids
What mineral is important in cell membranes?	Phosphorous

What does saturated refer to?	All carbons of a fatty acid are saturated with hydrogens so no double bonds
Double bonds are seen in what kind of FA?	Unsaturated
How are lipids transported in the blood?	Via lipoproteins
How many carbons in a short chain FA?	2–6
How many carbons in a medium chain FA?	8–10
How many carbons in a long chain FA?	16–22
Animal fat is a good source of what type of FA?	Saturated
Oleic, linoleic and alpha linolenic acids are examples of what type of FA?	Unsaturated
Hydrogenation of fatty acids produces what?	Cis and Trans fatty acids
What are 2 effects of trans-fatty acids on the body?	1. Interfere with essential fatty acid metabolism 2. Atherogenesis
What substance emulsifies FAs?	Bile
How do triglycerides cross the intestinal membrane?	They drop 2 fatty acids leaving one at the number 2 site on glycerol, cross membrane and get reformed on the other side
How do triglycerides travel in general circulation?	Via chylomicrons in the lymphatics and blood stream
Where does beta oxidation take place?	In the mitochondrion of all cells
What is the activated form of FA?	Acetyl-CoA
How is Acetyl-CoA transported into the mitochondrion?	Via carnitine
What co-enzyme is needed in the activation of FA into Acetyl-CoA?	Vitamin B5
What co-enzymes are needed in the beta-oxidation pathway?	Vitamin B2 as FAD Vitamin B3 as NAD

Where does FA synthesis take place?	In cytosol of all cells
What is the rate-limiting enzyme of FA synthesis?	Acetyl-CoA carboxylase
What is the immediate substrate for FA synthesis?	Acetyl-CoA
Acetyl-CoA carboxylase acts on Acetyl-CoA to produce what?	Malonyl-CoA
What co-enzyme is important for the production of Malonyl-CoA from Acetyl-CoA?	Biotin
What reducing agent is used in FA synthesis?	NADPH
How does Acetyl-CoA get out into the cytoplasm for FA synthesis?	Citrate leaves the mitochondrion and the action of citrate lyase forms Acetyl-CoA and oxaloacetate
What hormone activates Acetyl-CoA carboxylase?	Insulin
What is the end product of de novo FA synthesis?	Palmitate
What substance is the activated end product of lipogenesis and will cause feedback inhibition on Acetyl-CoA carboxylase?	Palmitoyl-CoA
What 3 tissues undergo lipogenesis?	Liver, skeletal muscle, and cardiac muscle
Where does chain elongation take place?	In the mitochondrion and smooth ER
Which tissues undergo de novo synthesis?	Liver and adipose cells
Where does do novo synthesis take place?	In the cytoplasm
What are the 3 Ketone Bodies?	Acetoacetate, acetone and beta hydroxybutarate
Ketone production takes place when which substance is low?	Oxaloacetate

In what tissue does ketone synthesis take place?	Liver
Where in the cell does ketone synthesis take place?	In the mitochondrial matrix
What is the fate of acetone?	It is usually exhaled
What is the fate of 3 hydroxybutarate?	It gets oxidized to acetoacetate
What 2 tissues can use acetoacetate?	Brain and skeletal muscle
What are the 2 essential fatty acids?	Linoleic acid Alpha linolenic acid
What is a good source of linoleic acid?	Vegetables, nuts and seeds
What is a good source for alpha-linolenic acid?	Flaxseeds
What is the name of the enzyme that converts linoleic and alpha-linolenic acids into their metabolites?	Delta-6-desaturase
Which EFA is omega-3?	Alpha-linolenic acid
Which EFA is omega-6?	Linoleic acid
Which FA is the precursor for pro-inflammatory, series 2 eicosanoids?	Arachadonic acid
Which EFA is precursor for series 1 eicosanoids?	Linoleic acid
Which EFA is precursor for series 3 eicosanoids?	Alpha-linolenic acid
Linoleic acid is converted by delta-6-desaturase into what fatty acid?	Gamma-linolenic acid
What are some good sources of gamma-linolenic acid?	Evening primrose oil, borage oil, blackcurrant oil
What important fatty acid, also known as 20:5(n-3) can alpha-linolenic acid be converted into?	Eicosapentaenoic acid

What is a good source of eicosapentaeinoic acid?	Cold water fish oils
What is the name of the enzyme that releases arachidonic acid from cell membranes?	Phospholipase A2
What is the name of the enzyme that converts arachadonic acid into prostaglandins?	Cyclooxygenase
What is the name of the enzyme that forms leukotrienes from arachadonic acid?	Lipoxygenase
What products inhibit phospholipase A2?	Corticosteroid anti-inflammatories
What product inhibits activity of cyclooxygenase?	NSAIDs
What hormone promotes the conversion of carbohydrates into triglycerides?	Insulin
What enzyme causes the release of fatty acids from triglycerides?	Hormone sensitive lipase
What are free fatty acids usually bound to in the blood?	Albumin
What hormone inhibits action of hormone sensitive lipase?	Insulin
What promotes hormone sensitive lipase?	Growth hormone, glucagon and Epi
Esterification is used in the forming of triglycerides from what 2 substances?	Acetyl-CoA and glycerol-6-phosphate
Free fatty acids are mobilized from what cell?	Adipose
What apoprotein marks HDL for hepatic uptake?	Aporotein E
How is dietary fat carried into the body?	In chylomicrons via the lacteals
Which tissues synthesize chylomicrons?	Mucosal cells of small intestine
Apoprotein A is found on what lipoprotein?	HDL

Which lipoprotein functions to carry triglycerides from the liver to extrahepatic tissue?	VLDL
Which lipoprotein functions to carry cholesterol from liver to extrahepatic tissue?	LDL
Which apoprotein allows for uptake of cholesterol by cells?	Apoprotein B
Chylomicron remnants are formed from the action of which enzyme?	Apoprotein lipase
What enzyme facilitates cholesterol transfer to HDL from tissues?	Lecithin-cholesterol acyltransferase
What apoprotein activates Lecithin-cholesterol acyltransferase?	Apoprotein A on HDL
Which transfer protein facilitates transfer of cholesterol from LDL and VLDL to HDL?	Cholesterol transfer protein

Basic Steroid Biochemistry

In which tissues does cholesterol synthesis take place?	Liver and intestines
Where in the cell does cholesterol synthesis take place?	Cytoplasm
What is the precursor for cholesterol synthesis?	Acetyl-CoA
What pathway is the greatest producer of Acetyl-CoA?	Beta-oxidation
What is the rate-limiting, regulatory enzyme of cholesterol synthesis?	HMG-CoA reductase
What hormone promotes the action of HMG-CoA reductase?	Insulin
What are the 2 significant intermediates in cholesterol synthesis?	HMG-CoA and mevalonate
What is the function of cholesterol?	Membrane fluidity, precursor to all steroid hormones

What type of fatty acids increase cholesterol? Which decrease it?	Increase: Saturated fats Decrease: Unsaturated fats
What metabolite is formed from mevalonate?	CoQ_{10}
What 2 hormones are released in response to fatty chyme reaching the duodenum?	Secretin and Cholecystokinin
What hormone secreted from the intestines is responsible for increasing bile production in the Liver and stimulating bile secretion from the liver?	Secretin
What hormone produced by the intestines stimulates the hepatopancreatic sphincter to relax, stimulates secretion of pancreatic juices, and cause the gallbladder to contract and release bile?	Cholecystokinin (CCK)
What role do bile salts play in fat absorption?	They emulsify fats to enhance their absorption
What 2 substance acts as a conjugating agents to convert bile acids into bile salts?	Taurine and glycine
What enzyme is the rate limiting step in bile acid formation?	7-alpha-hydroxylase
What vitamin is needed for the activity of 7-alpha-hydroxylase?	Vitamin C
What are the 2 primary bile acids?	Cholic acid Chenodeoxycholic acid
What are the 2 secondary bile acids?	Deoxycholic acid Lithocholic acid
Where are bile acids formed?	Liver and intestines
Where are bile acids stored?	Gallbladder
Where does bile acid reabsorption take place?	Ileum
What are the 2 functions of bile acids?	Fat emulsification Cholesterol excretion

GASTROINTESTINAL

Testosterone is produced in which tissues?	Adrenal cortex, testes
Estrone and estradiol are produced in which tissue?	Ovaries and small amount in adrenal cortex
DHEA, progesterone, cortisol and aldosterone are produced in which tissue?	Adrenal cortex
What is precursor for steroid hormones?	Cholesterol
What vitamin is needed for steroid hormone production?	Vitamin C

Basic Amino Acids and Protein Biochemistry

Tryptophan is a precursor for what neurotransmitters?	Serotonin and melatonin
The reaction of tryptophan to serotonin requires what vitamin as a co-factor?	Vitamin B6 (pyridoxine)
Tryptophan can also be turned into what molecule?	Niacin
Tyrosine is the precursor for which three neurotransmitters?	Dopamine, norepinephrine and epinephrine
What is the rate limiting cofactor in the conversion of tryptophan to 5-hydroxytryptophan, phenylalanine to tyrosine, and tyrosine to dopamine?	5-methyltetrahydrofolate (active folic acid)
What is the rate-limiting enzyme for the production of L-DOPA (and therefore catecholamines in general) from tyrosine?	Tyrosine hydroxolase
What factors inhibit and promote the activity of tyrosine hydroxolase?	Promotes: Cold, stress Inhibits: Norepi
What vitamin is needed as a cofactor for the production of norepi from dopamine?	Vitamin C
What is the name of the enzyme that breaks down Norepi and epinephrine?	Monoamineoxidase (MAO)
What is the breakdown product of MAO's action on Norepi and Epi?	Vanillmandelic acid (VMA)

What are the 3 branched chain amino acids?	Valine, isoleucine and leucine
Post-translational modification of proline and lysine to form hydroxylysine and hydroxyproline in collagen formation requires which vitamin?	Vitamin C
Which 3 amino acids can be post-translationally modified by phosphorylation?	Serine Threonine Tyrosine
GABA (Gamma-aminobutyric acid) is formed from what amino acid?	Glutamate/glutamic acid
The conversion of glutamic acid to GABA requires what vitamin as a cofactor?	Vitamin B6 (pyridoxine)
Histamine is formed from what amino acid?	Histidine
Which amino acid is the main methyl donor in the body?	Methionine
What are the 6 amino acids that can be catabolized by skeletal muscle?	Valine Aspartic acid Leucine Asparagine Isoleucine Glutamic acid
What are the 3 amino acids that make up the tripeptide glutathione?	Cysteine, glycine and glutamic acid
What are the 2 initial precursors for heme synthesis?	Glycine and Succinyl-Coa
What 2 amino acids form cysteine?	Glycine and arginine
What amino acid is the main transporter of nitrogen (ammonia) in the blood?	Glutamine
Alanine can be converted into what substance?	Pyruvate
What amino acid is a major component of actin and myosin? What form does it take?	Histidine in the form of 3-methyl-histidine

What type of bond holds together the amino acid sequence of peptides?	Covalent
What are the only 2 sulphur-containing dietary amino acids?	Methionine and cysteine
What 2 bonds hold a secondary protein structure?	Disulfide and weak
3-D folding of proteins is seen in which structure?	Tertiary
2 or more single polypeptide chains bonded by weak bonds is called what?	Quaternary structure
The heme molecule is an example of what type of protein structure?	Quaternary
2 Cysteine residues can form what type of bond?	Disulfide
A water-soluble protein is known as what?	A globular protein
Hydrogen bonds, salt bridges (or ionic attraction) and hydrophobic interactions are classified as what type of bond?	Weak
Atoms that share 1 or more electrons are bonded by what type of bond?	Covalent
What are the 10 essential amino acids?	Threonine, lysine, valine, leucine, methionine, tryptophan, phenylalanine, histidine, isoleucine, arginine.
The removal of an alpha-amino group from an amino acid is the first stage in amino acid catabolism and is known as what?	Transamination
Catabolism of amino acids uses what 2 types of reaction?	Oxidative deamination and transamination
The effect of transamination reactions is to collect the amino groups from all the other amino acids in the form of only one amino acid, which one?	Glutamate

Transaminases require what vitamin as a co-factor?	Vitamin B6, pyridoxine
In which tissues does oxidative deamination occur?	In the liver and kidneys
In what part of the cell does oxidative deamination take place?	The mitochondria
What is the main amino acid to undergo oxidative deamination?	Glutamate
What is the main enzyme in oxidative deamination?	Glutamine dehydrogenase
Which amino acid is present in blood in the highest levels?	Glutamine. It is the major carrier of amino groups. It allows transport of toxic nitrogen in a non-toxic form from extrahepatic tissues to the liver.
Glutamine synthetase is the enzyme that catalyzes the reaction of glutamate into glutamine. Its levels are especially high in which tissue?	The brain, as it is especially sensitive to ammonia.
Which amino acid transfers ammonia from muscle to the liver?	Alanine
Urea is formed from what 2 molecules?	CO_2 and ammonia
Where does the urea cycle take place?	The liver
How is the urea cycle regulated?	Substrate availability, i.e. dietary protein
Where do the 2 nitrogen atoms in urea come from?	One from ammonia and one from aspartate
Which Krebs cycle intermediate is produced by the urea cycle?	Fumarate
What are the 4 major constituents of urine?	Urea, ammonia, creatinine and uric acid
What is the role of HCL in protein digestion?	To denature the protein and provide optimal pH for pepsinogen conversion to pepsin
What enzyme has optimum activity at pH2?	Pepsisinogen which is converted into pepsin

What three aromatic amino acids have their peptide bonds hydrolyzed by pepsin?	Tyrosine, phenylalanine and tryptophan
Enterokinase is the enzyme that activates which zymogen released by the pancreas?	Trypsinogen
Which enzyme activates all the other zymogens released by the pancreas?	Trypsin
What is the overall fate of proteins that we eat?	They form free amino acids and enter the liver via the portal blood supply
What is the role of brush border enzymes in protein digestion?	They break down the smaller peptides to release free amino acids which are transported across the epithelial cells and enter blood capillaries
Which bonds need to be broken for a protein to become denatured?	Weak and disulfide bonds

Basic Nucleic Acid and Genetic Biochemistry

What are the building blocks of nucleic acids called?	Nucleotides
What are the 3 characteristic components of a nucleotide?	Nitrogenous base (purine or pyrimidine), a pentose sugar (ribose or deoxyribose) and a phosphate group.
A nucleotide minus the phosphate group is known as what?	A nucleoside
What kind of bond joins nucleic acids in RNA and DNA?	$3',5'$--phosphodiester bonds.
Where does purine and pyrimidine synthesis occur?	In the liver
What other tissue produces significant quantities of purine and pyrimidine?	The brain
What metabolic pathway produces ribose residues for nucleic acid synthesis?	Hexose monophosphate shunt
What molecule is the precursor for adenine and guanine?	IMP or inositol monophosphate

What molecule is the precursor for cytosine, uracil, and thyamine?	UMP or uridine monophosphate
What are the precursors for pyrimidine synthesis?	Glutamine and CO_2
What is an important co-enzyme in purine and pyrimidine synthesis?	Folic acid
In de novo synthesis of purines what is the starting material?	Ribose-5-phosphate
What does DNA stand for?	Deoxyribonucleic Acid
What makes RNA different from DNA?	Smaller strand of genetic information No de-oxy sugar Contains uracil, not thymine
What are the 3 different types of RNA?	mRNA- Messanger RNA tRNA- Transport RNA rRNA- Ribosomal RNA
What is the function of tRNA?	To bring the correct amino acid in line with the correct codon
What is the function of mRNA?	It carries the genetic sequence information from the genes to the ribosome to be coded
What is the function of rRNA?	Aids transfer RNA in translation
Making RNA from a DNA template is known as what?	Transcription
Regarding RNA and DNA what does translation mean?	It the process by which the information from mRNA is decoded and used to assemble the polypeptide
What factors can separate DNA strands?	An increase in temperature Changing the salt concentration around it
Three consecutive base pairs are known as what?	A codon
What are the four nucleotide bases that make up DNA?	Adenine, Guanine, Cytosine, Thymine.

What are the 2 pyrimidines found in DNA?	Cytosine and Thymine
What are the 2 pyrimidines found in RNA?	Cytosine and Uracil
What are the 2 purines in RNA and DNA?	Adenine and Guanine
Adenine pairs with which other nucleotide bases?	Thymine, Uracil
Cytosine pairs with which base?	Guanine
Where does pyrimidine and purine catabolism occur mainly?	The Liver
In RNA what nucleotide base stands in for thymine?	Uracil
Purine degradation generates what molecule?	Uric acid
Pyrimidines are degrade into what molecules?	Carbon dioxide and water
What is the name for the last enzyme in the production of uric acid from purines?	Xanthine oxidase
What mineral is needed as a cofactor in the conversion of purine into uric acid?	Molybdenum

Basic Enzyme Biochemistry

What do enzymes do in chemical reactions?	They lower the activation energy of a reaction and increase the rate of the reaction
What 2 things affect enzyme activity?	pH and temperature
The synthesis of an enzyme needed for breakdown of a certain substrate is initiated by the presence of that substrate is known as what?	Induction

Modulation of an enzyme by the non-covalent binding of a specific metabolite at a site other than the active site is an example of what?	Allosteric activity
Molecules that must undergo cleavage reactions in order to become active are known as what?	Zymogens
Substances that hold an enzyme in certain configurations so that it can function are known as what?	Co-factors or co-enzymes
Phosphorylation or dephosphorylation of an enzyme is an example of what?	Covalent modification
An enzyme bound to its co-enzyme is known as what?	An holozyme
Multiple forms of an enzyme that catalyze the same reaction but differ from each other in amino acid sequence, substrate affinity and regulatory properties are known as what?	Isozymes

Basic Nutritional and Clinical Biochemistry

Vitamin B1 is known as what?	Thiamin
Vitamin B2 is known as what?	Riboflavin
Vitamin B3 is known as what?	Niacin or nicotinic acid
Vitamin B5 is known as what?	Pantothenic acid
Vitamin B6 is known as what	Pyridoxine
Vitamin B12 is known as what?	Cobalamin
What is the active form of B1/thiamin called?	Thiamin pyrophosphate
What mineral is often required in reactions involving vitamin B1/thiamin as a cofactor?	Magnesium
Transketolase in the hexose shunt requires what vitamin?	Vitamin B1 (thiamin)

Oxidative carboxylation in the pyruvate dehydrogenase complex needs what vitamin?	Vitamin B1 (thiamin), vitamin B2 (FAD), vitamin B3 (NAD), and vitamin B5 (CoA)
What vitamin plays a role in transamination reactions?	Vitamin B6 (pyridoxine)
Where is vitamin B1 (thiamin) absorbed?	Jejunum or ileum
FAD and FMN are active constituents of what vitamin?	Vitamin B2 (riboflavin)
Where is vitamin B2 (riboflavin) absorbed?	Duodenum or jejunum
What vitamins are used in oxidation-reduction reactions/ electron transfer reactions (dehydrogenase enzymes)?	Vitamin B3 (niacin) and vitamin B2 (riboflavin)
What form of niacin is used in synthesis pathways?	NADPH
NAD and NADH are the oxidized and reduced forms of what vitamin?	Vitamin B3 (niacin)
What amino acid can form niacin?	Tryptophan
Where is pantothenic acid absorbed?	Jejunum
Which vitamin is essential for reactions using CoA?	Vitamin B5 (pantothenic acid)
Pyridoxal phosphate is the active form of what vitamin?	Vitamin B6 (pyridoxine)
What mineral is needed to activate vitamin B6?	Magnesium
Which vitamin serves as CO_2 carrier in carboxylation reactions?	Biotin
Which vitamin is essential for nucleotide synthesis and for single carbon transfer?	Folic acid
What vitamin is needed as a co-factor to activate folic acid?	Vitamin B12 (cobalamin)
What is the first active form of B12?	Methylcobalamin

List some of the biochemical activities of Vitamin C	a. Reducing agent b. Co-factor for hydroxylation reactions eg. proline, dopamine and norep/epi synthesis c. Carnitine synthesis d. Enhances iron mobilization e. Bile acid formation f. Influence on cholesterol metabolism
What is the active form of vitamin A in the blood?	Retinol
What is the active form of vitamin A in the eyes?	Retinal
What is the active form of vitamin A in epithelial cells?	Retinoic acid
This mineral is a constituent of DNA and RNA.	Phosphorous
Which vitamin is a co-factor in post synthetic modification of proteins via a carboxylation reaction, which allows for the chelation of calcium?	Vitamin K
What is the storage form of vitamin A in the liver?	Retinyl palmitate
Where is vitamin A absorbed?	Lumen of S.I.
Which of the active forms of vitamin D increases serum calcium?	$1,25\text{-}(OH_2)D_3$
Which of the active forms of vitamin D lowers serum calcium?	$24,25\text{-}(OH_2)D_3$
Where are the inactive metabolites of vitamin D converted to active form?	Kidney primarily, also in neurons, leukocytes, and other peripheral tissues
Which hormone plays a role in activating vitamin D?	Parathyroid hormone
Where is vitamin E stored?	Adipose tissue

Fat soluble-vitamins, like Vit E, depend on what for their absorption from the intestinal lumen?	Pancreatic esterases and bile salts
What converts 7-hydroxycholesterol into cholecalciferol?	Sunlight on the skin
Beta-carotene is a precursor to what vitamin?	Vitamin A
What vitamin is required for the biosynthesis of clotting factors?	Vitamin K
What is the active form of vitamin K?	Hydroquinone
Which mineral is important for energy-producing reactions?	Phosphorous
The production of osteocalcin is dependent on what vitamin?	Vitamin K
What mineral is important for clotting?	Calcium
This mineral, once it is attached to a substance, traps it inside the cell.	Phosphorous
All the reactions using ATP use this mineral as a cofactor.	Magnesium
This mineral activates a number of B vitamins.	Magnesium
Which mineral is the most abundant intracellularly?	Potassium
What mineral is in cytochromes?	Iron
Which mineral is an insulin cofactor?	Chromium
Which mineral is a part of glutathione peroxidase?	Selenium
Which mineral is a part of vitamin B12?	Cobalt
Which mineral is important for the biosynthesis of thyroid hormones?	Iodine

Which mineral is needed for cholesterol synthesis?	Manganese
What is the blood transport form of iron?	Transferrin
What is the main storage form of iron?	Ferritin
What stores excess iron?	Hemosidirin
What substance is protective in that it keeps iron away from bacteria?	Lactoferrin
What are the 3 sources of glucose in the body?	Gluconeogenesis, dietary, and glycogen breakdown
How is glucose transported in the body?	Free
Glycogen is formed in all tissues but especially which 3?	Liver, cardiac and skeletal muscle
Complete oxidation means what?	The complete breakdown of carbohydrates, proteins or fatty acids into ATP, CO_2 and water.
Incomplete oxidation or anaerobic glycolysis forms what substance?	Lactate
Excess glucose is converted to what?	Fatty acids especially in adipose and liver
What are the 2 sources of blood triglycerides?	Diet and synthesis by liver and mucosal cells of intestine
How are dietary triglycerides transported?	By chylomicrons
How do triglycerides travel from liver into the blood?	Via VLDLs
True or false: Triglycerides can cross membranes.	False, they need lipoprotein to cross membranes
What kind of bonds does lipoprotein lipase break?	Ester bonds
What is the fate of triglycerides?	They get broken down by lipoprotein lipase and free fatty acids are released
How are free fatty acids transported?	Via albumin in the blood

GASTROINTESTINAL

What are the 2 sources of blood cholesterol?	Diet and synthesis by liver
Blood levels of cholesterol are mainly affected by what?	Liver synthesis
What are the 2 main carrier proteins in the blood?	Albumin Globulin
What enzyme catalyzes the conversion of lactate into pyruvate?	LDH (Lactate Dehydrogenase)
How many LDH isoenzymes are there?	5
What enzyme catalyzes the conversion of creatine into creatine phosphate?	CPK (Creatine Phosphokinase)
What enzyme transfers an amino group from alanine to alpha-ketoglutartae?	ALT or SGPT
What enzyme transfers an amino group from glutamate to oxaloacetate to form aspartate?	AST or SGOT
What are the major sources for SGOT/AST?	Cardiac tissue Liver Skeletal muscle RBCs
What are the major sources for SGPT/ALT?	Highest concentration in the liver Also found in the heart, skeletal muscle, and RBCs.
Glucokinase, hexokinase, phosphofructokinase and pyruvate kinase are found in which pathway?	Glycolysis
Which enzyme, when turned on, allows Acetyl-CoA to be used for gluconeogenesis?	Pyruvate Carboxylase
Which enzyme, when turned on, allows Acetyl-CoA to be used for ATP production?	Pyruvate dehydrogenase complex

Glucose-6-phosphatase, fructose 1,6-bisphosphatase and pyruvate carboxykinase are found in what pathway?	Gluconeogenic pathway
Carnitine is found in which pathway?	Lipolysis/beta oxidation
Palmitoyl-CoA is found in which pathway?	Lipogenesis
Malonyl-CoA is found in which pathway?	Lipogenesis
Acetyl-CoA carboxylase is found in which pathway?	Lipogenesis
Ubiquinone and cytochromes are found in which pathway?	Electron transport chain
Citrate lyase is found in which pathway?	Lipogenesis
Delta-6-desaturase is found in which pathway?	Eicosanoid production pathway
Phospholipase A2 is found in which pathway?	Eicosanoid production from arachadonic acid
Cyclooxygenase is found in which pathway?	In the prostaglandin synthesis pathway from arachadonic acid
Hmg-CoA reductase is found in which pathway?	Cholesterol synthesis
7 alpha hydroxylase is found in which pathway?	Bile synthesis
Mevalonate is found in which pathway?	Cholesterol synthesis

Pathology

What bacteria causes severe gastroenteritis and can be caught from shellfish?	*Yersinia enterocolitica* *Vibrio parahemolyticus* *Salmonella typhi*
What organisms can exist chronically in the gall bladder?	*Salmonella typhi, Giardia lamblia*

GASTROINTESTINAL

What organism, having many animal reservoirs produces endotoxin and is a common cause of food poisoning in the USA?	*Salmonella enterides*
What causes bacillary dysentry?	*Shigella dysenteriae*
Compare *Salmonella* and *Staphylococcus* food poisoning in terms of incubation and explain why?	*Staphyloccus*: 4–8 h because it produces exotoxin *Salmonella*: 10–28 h because the cells have to die and start producing exotoxin
Rice water stool is associated with infection by what organism?	*Vibrio cholerae*
What organism causes infectious jaundice?	*Leptospira interrogans*
What organism contracted from raw milk causes bloody diarrhea and can mimic appendicitis?	*Campylobacter jejuni*
What organism is implicated in causing peptic ulcers?	*Helicobacter pylori*
What happens when salicylates are given during viral illness?	Reye's syndrome
What are the most common potential complications of Reye's syndrome?	Liver damage Encephalopathy
Which age group is most affected with hepatitis A virus (HAV)?	Children
How is HAV transmitted?	Fecal-oral route
Which immunoglobulin rises early in the HAV infection?	IgM
What is the incubation period for HAV?	3–4 weeks
What symptoms are common in early hepatitis A?	Fever Jaundice Nausea
What are some of the other signs of HAV infection?	Dark-colored urine, Clay colored stools, Elevation of serum liver enzymes

What are the three known methods of contracting HBV?	Blood Perinatally Sexual contact
What is the incubation period for HBV?	10–12 days
What symptoms commonly occur in HBV infection?	Fever Fatigue Nausea Jaundice with hepatomegaly Arthralgia Arthritis
What serum antigen of HBV tends to rise 1–6 weeks before clinical symptoms?	HBsAg (surface antigen)
What serum antigen of HBV occurs during active infection?	HBeAg (e antigen)
What serum antibody against HBV appears weeks after recovery?	Anti-HBsAb (anti-surface antibody)
What serum antibody against HBV appears at onset of clinical symptoms or suggests current or past infection?	Anti-HBcAb (anti-core antibody)
What serum antibody against HBV suggests low risk of infectivity and shows a good chance of avoiding chronic liver disease?	Anti-HBeAb (anti-e antibody)
Why does HBV have a potential carrier state?	Viral DNA is integrated in the chromosome of the host cell
What segment of the public has a high rate of hepatitis C virus (HCV) infection?	IV drug users, transfusion or blood product recipients prior to 1992
The delta particle is associated with what disease?	Hepatitis D
What is the transmission route for each type of viral hepatitis?	Hepatitis A (HAV) — fecal-oral route Hepatitis B (HBV) — sexual and parenteral routes Hepatitis C (HCV) — arenteral route Hepatitis D (HDV) — sexual and parenteral routes Hepatitis E (HEV) — fecal-oral route

Which type of hepatitis occurs concurrently with another hepatitis infection?	Hepatitis D requires concurrent infection with hepatitis B
Which types of hepatitis may progress to chronic hepatitis?	Hepatitis B Hepatitis C
What is the most common cause of transfusion-mediated hepatitis?	Hepatitis C
Alcoholic hepatitis involves what changes in the liver?	Infiltration by neutrophils Focal liver cell necrosis Presence of Mallory bodies Fatty changes in the liver Fibrosis leading to central venous obstruction
What type of inflammation of the gums may occur in patients with compromised immune systems?	Acute necrotizing ulcerative gingivitis (trench mouth)
Chronic gingivitis may lead to what condition?	Periodontitis
Candidal stomatitis is also known by what other names?	Thrush Oral candidiasis Moniliasis
What are Koplik's spots?	Lesions that appear on the oral mucosa early in measles
What causes most inflammation of the esophagus?	Gastric acid reflux
What causes Barrett's esophagus?	Long-standing reflux esophagitis causes gastric metaplasia of the lower esophagus, creating susceptibility to peptic ulceration, esophageal stricture, and adenocarcinoma. Some argue that Barrett's is a completely different phenotype of GERD not related to long-standing disease.
What are predisposing factors to esophageal cancer?	Nitrosamines from smoked meats Alcoholism Smoking Esophagitis

What are the two types of chronic gastritis?	Fundal (type A) gastritis Antral (type B) gastritis
What symptoms occur with acute gastritis?	Pain, nausea, vomiting, possible occult blood
What occurs with fundal (type A) gastritis?	Decrease or absence of gastric acid production from failure or destruction of parietal cells
Chronic gastritis is associated with what type of infection?	Helicobacter pylori infection
What causes peptic ulcers?	Imbalance between acid secretion and mucous barrier protection, leading to erosion of stomach or duodenal mucosa
What contributes to duodenal ulcers?	Hypersecretion of gastric acid and pepsin
When does the pain begin with duodenal ulcers?	90 minutes to 3 hours after eating, relieved by food
When does the pain begin with gastric ulcers?	Within 30 minutes after eating, not relieved by food
What problems may occur with hypochlorhydria or achlorhydria?	a. Difficulty digesting protein b. Food sensitivities c. Constipation d. Gas and bloating e. Heartburn f. Mineral deficiencies
What is a hiatal hernia?	Part of the stomach slides through the esophageal hiatus of the diaphragm
What is most commonly true of gastric cancer?	a. It is usually adenocarcinoma b. It is more common in Japan (50% of all cancers) c. It usually occurs after 50 years of age
What is intussusception?	A proximal segment of bowel telescopes into a distal segment, causing obstruction
What is volvulus?	Twisting of part of the GI tract, often causing obstruction

What causes gastroenteritis?	Ingesting food containing bacteria that: 1. Contain preformed toxins, i.e., *Clostridiumbotulinum, S. aureus* 2. Form a toxin, i.e., *Vibrio cholerae, E.coli, Campylobacter jejuni* 3. Invade intestinal cells, i.e., *Salmonella, Shigella, E. coli, Yersinia enterocolitica,* rotavirus
What is typically found in Crohn's disease?	Transmural skip lesions and non-caseous granulomas of the terminal ileum or colon
What causes celiac disease?	Hypersensitivity reaction to gliadin causing destruction of mucosal villi of the jejunum
What is found in diverticulosis?	Multiple diverticula in the sigmoid colon without inflammation
What is diverticulitis?	Inflamed diverticula, which may cause perforation, peritonitis, abscesses, and bowel stenosis
What predisposes one to hemorrhoids?	Low-fiber diet
What are the two types of colitis?	Chronic ulcerative Microbial
What is typically found in colitis?	Continuous ulcerous and inflamed lesions in the rectum and descending colon causing bloody diarrhea with mucous
What is the most common cause of pseudomembranous colitis?	Overgrowth of Clostridium difficile
Hamartomatous polyps most often occur in what syndrome?	Peutz-Jeghers syndrome
What is the most common form of polyp?	Tubular adenomas, which are small and pedunculated and contain malignant foci
What is believed to be the cause of acute appendicitis?	Obstruction of the lumen by a hard mass of feces, a fecalith, which causes bacterial infection and purulent exudate

What are the symptoms of acute appendicitis?	a. Anorexia b. Nausea c. Abdominal pain, most commonly in the right lower quadrant
What is a test used to detect colorectal cancer?	Fecal occult blood screening
Chronic pancreatitis is most commonly associated with what condition?	Alcoholism
What are common symptoms of pancreatic cancer?	Abdominal pain radiating to the back Anorexia Weight loss Migratory thrombophlebitis
Chronic liver failure is most commonly associated with what conditions?	Alcoholic cirrhosis Chronic viral hepatitis
What enzymes are elevated in acute liver failure?	Serum alanine aminotransferase (ALT) Aspartate aminotransferase (AST) Lactate dehydrogenase (LDH)
What is a common tumor marker for hepatocellular carcinoma?	Serum alpha-fetoprotein (AFP)
What may happen with portal hypertension?	Splenomegaly Ascites Hemorrhoids Esophageal varices
What is formed from the normal or abnormal destruction of red blood cells and can cause pigmentation of the skin?	Bilirubin
Excess bilirubin is associated with what condition?	Jaundice
What causes obstructive jaundice?	Conjugated (direct) bilirubin from obstruction, i.e., gallstones, tumors, and strictures; cirrhosis; hepatitis; drugs; and pregnancy
What is the most dangerous cause of jaundice?	Unconjugated (indirect) bilirubin from hemolysis

Cirrhosis is often associated with which type of cancer?

Hepatocellular carcinoma

What are common signs and symptoms of cholecystitis?

Nausea and vomiting
Fever
Right upper quadrant and epigastric pain
Leukocytosis

Hematopoietic System

Embryology

Angioblasts form from what?	Mesoderm
Angioblasts form what as they cluster?	Blood islands
The blood islands fuse together to form what?	A primordial vascular network
Hemocytoblasts arise from what?	Core cells within these islands
Blood formation occurs at what week?	Week 5

Anatomy

Where in bone marrow are erythrocytes produced?	Within the blood sinusoids of the red bone marrow
Explain the path by which a hemocytoblast becomes an erythrocyte	Hemocytoblast → proerythroblast → early erythroblast → late erythroblast → normoblast → reticulocyte → erythrocyte
In which of these stages of development is the nucleus detached and released from the cell?	The normoblast
Which protein is responsible for the biconcave shape of erythrocytes?	Spectrin, which gives them their flexibility
Which B vitamins are key in the production of erythrocytes?	Vitamin B12 and Folate

What happens to older erythrocytes?	They lose their flexibility and become trapped and break in small capillaries like in the spleen
After erythrocytes break apart what happens?	They are engulfed by macrophages
What happens to the parts of the erythrocyte?	a. The heme is broken off the globin b. The globin is broken down into amino acids c. The heme is degraded into bilirubin d. the iron is stored as ferritin or hemosiderin
How much of plasma is water?	90%
What solutes are carried in plasma?	Proteins, cellular by-products (ex: urea), metabolic nutrients (ex: amino acids), electrolytes (ex: sodium), and respiratory gases (ex: oxygen)
Which protein is the most abundant in plasma?	Albumin

Physiology

What are the 2 cell types that form blood cells?	Erythrocytes (red blood cells) Leukocytes (white cells)
What are the 3 main plasma proteins?	Albumin Globulins Fibrinogen
What is the major blood electrolyte?	Sodium
Where does erythropoesis take place?	In the bone marrow
Cessation of bleeding is known as what?	Hemostasis
What is role of platelets in hemostasis?	They stick to the injured site causing a platelet plug
What makes up a clot?	Platelet plug plus fibrin
What do you call a clot that includes RBCs?	A thrombus

Vitamin K is important for which factors?	II, VII, IX and X
What initiates the intrinsic pathway of the blood coagulation cascade?	Blood coming in contact with exposed collagen of the damaged tissue
What mineral is needed for proper clotting?	Calcium
What is the insoluble substance that precipitates out at injury site?	Fibrin
What substance dissolves clots?	Plasmin
What substance cleaves fibrinogen into fibrin?	Thrombin
Which hormone stimulates erythrocyte formation and from what organ is it excreted?	The kidneys secret erythropoietin to stimulate red blood cell production
What functions does blood play in the body?	Distributing oxygen and removing cellular waste, moving hormones, preventing illness, and maintaining body temperature, fluid, and pH

Biochemistry

What substance, when bound to heme, weakens the oxygen/heme bond and causes release of oxygen?	2,3-bisphosphoglycerate (2,3-BPG)
Thiamine is also needed for what transketolase reaction?	The hexose monophosphate shunt
What role does the hexose monophosphate shunt play in erythrocytes?	It produces NADPH which keeps glutathione in a reduced state
What can bind to hemoglobin?	O_2, CO_2 and CO, H+, 2,3-bisphosphoglycerate
What amino acid is needed to maintain the functionality and structure of the hemoglobin?	Histidine
What are the three functions of hemoglobin?	Transport oxygen Transport carbon dioxide Act as a blood buffer

What 2 substances are the starting materials for heme synthesis?	Succinyl-CoA and glycine
What do they form?	Delta aminolevulenic acid
What is the regulatory enzyme in heme synthesis?	Delta-aminolevulenic acid synthase (ALAS)
The formation of porphobilinogen from Delta aminolevulenic acid is catalyzed by what enzyme?	Delta-aminolevulenic dehydrogenase (ALAD)
What substance inhibits ALAD?	Lead
What mineral is incorporated into heme?	Iron
Where does this take place?	In the mitochondrion
Where in the body does heme synthesis take place?	In the bone marrow
Congenital deficiencies of certain enzymes in the heme synthesis can cause what?	Porphyrias
In what other substances is heme found?	Myoglobin, cytochromes
Where does catabolism of heme take place?	First the spleen, then the liver and finally the intestines. It also occurs in the bone marrow.
What breaks down heme during tissue damage?	Macrophages
What is the first substance produced by heme catabolism?	Biliverdin
Biliverdin is converted into what molecule?	Bilirubin
Where is bilirubin conjugated?	In the liver
How is bilirubin excreted?	In the bile
Bacteria in the gut convert some of the bilirubin into what substance?	Urobilinogen
What is the fate of urobilinogen?	It is reabsorbed, transported to the kidneys and converted to urobilin and excreted

What are the 2 excretory pathways for heme catabolism?	Feces and urine
What role does H+ binding to hemoglobin have?	It induces hemoglobin to unload its bound oxygen and helps buffer blood pH

Pathology

What is the vector for malaria?	*Anopheles* spp. mosquitoes
What do *Plasmodium* spp. cause?	Malaria
Which X-linked disorder is associated with a 99% loss of Factor VIII?	Hemophilia A
What does anemia cause in tissues?	Hypoxia (low oxygen)
What are general signs and symptoms of anemia?	1. Shortness of breath (dyspnea) with exertion 2. Fatigue 3. Lightheadedness or dizziness 4. Ringing in the ears (tinnitus) 5. Headache
What may result from long-term anemia?	1. Pallor 2. Increased heart rate (tachycardia) 3. Systolic ejection murmur 4. Orthostatic hypotension
What causes iron-deficiency anemia?	1. Chronic blood loss 2. Increased need for blood and oxygen 3. Decreased iron intake from poor absorption or dietary deficiency
What causes macrocytic anemia?	1. Vitamin B12 or folic acid deficiency 2. Malabsorption
Hemophilia is a genetic absence of what substances?	Hemophilia A: Factor VIII Hemophilia B: Factor IX
What are the symptoms of macrocytic anemia?	Glossitis, weight loss, peripheral neuropathy, depression and paranoia
What causes pernicious anemia?	Lack of intrinsic factor secreted by parietal cells of the stomach

What are the two specific symptoms of hemolysis?

1. Jaundice, from unconjugated bilirubin in the blood
2. Hemosiderosis, the deposition of iron

What causes red blood cell hemolysis?

1. Mechanical trauma to cells
2. Complement induced damage
3. Extravascular hemolysis

What are the most common forms of thalassemia in the Mediterranean and the United States?

Beta-thalasemmias

What are the most common forms of thalassemia in Southeast Asia?

Alpha-thalassemias

What is hereditary spherocytosis?

A genetic defect affecting northern Europeans in which spherical red blood cells become trapped in the spleen and destroyed

What is Glucose-6-Phosphate Dehydrogenase Deficiency?

It is an X-linked disorder that causes hemolytic anemia with oxidative stress

What causes aplastic anemia?

1. Toxic exposure, such as radiation
2. Chemicals
3. Therapeutic drugs
4. Viral infection
5. Idiopathic causes

What is polycythemia vera?

Polycythemia vera is a myeloproliferative disorder in which there is an increase in circulating red blood cells caused by neoplastic clonal proliferation in the marrow

What are the characteristics of acute forms of leukemia?

Acute leukemias have more poorly differentiated blast cells circulating

What are the characteristics of chronic forms of leukemia?

Chronic forms of leukemias have more differentiated cells in circulation and are diagnosed more frequently in older adults

What is a common laboratory finding in the diagnosis of chronic myelogenous leukemia?

Philadelphia chromosome

What are the characteristics of multiple myeloma?	1. Malignant neoplasm of B-lymphocytes 2. Affects 50–60 year olds 3. Punched out, lytic lesions in bone causing bone pain and fractures 4. Hypercalcemia from resorbed bone 5. Bacterial infections 6. Presence of Bence Jones proteins and renal failure
What is the name of the multi-nucleated giant cells found in Hodgkin's lymphoma?	Reed-Sternberg cells
What type of lymphoma affecting B-cells has an African and an American form?	Non-Hodgkin's lymphoma (Burkitt's lymphoma)
What is the most common hereditary clotting problem?	von Willebrand's Disease
Vitamin K is required for the synthesis of what clotting factors in the coagulation cascade?	Factors II (prothrombin), VII, IX, and X
What is the most common cause of abnormal bleeding?	Thrombocytopenia
What is thrombocytopenia?	A fall in platelets to below 70,000/μL, for which there are many potential causes. These include bone marrow damage, congenital problems, nutritional deficiencies, or increased destruction of platelets.
When does disseminated intravascular coagulation (DIC) occur?	After uncontrolled activation of clotting factors and fibrinolytic enzymes, often following major tissue damage from burns, sepsis, or complications of pregnancy.

Immunological System

Embryology

From what does the thymus arise?	The third Pharyngeal pouch
What tissue forms the cortex and medulla of thymus?	The cortex is formed from the ectoderm and the medulla is formed from the endoderm
What happens next?	The stroma tissue is populated with lymphocyte presursors from bone marrow
The spleen arises from which germ line?	Mesoderm
What are present in the spleen by the first trimester?	Macrophages
True or False: The spleen is capable of hematopoiesis during fetal life.	True, as well as after birth
What germ layer forms the bone marrow?	Mesoderm
Before bone marrow develops where are blood cells formed?	They start being produced in the yolk sac, then the liver takes over, and lastly the spleen handles the responsibility till the bone marrow matures.

Anatomy

Where is the thymus located?	In the upper anterior thorax just above the heart
At what age is the thymus fully developed by?	By birth
The involution of the thymus is almost complete by what age?	30 years of age
True or false: The thymus receives lymph.	False, the only route of access by cells is via blood
Describe the anatomy of the thymus	It is divided in the cortex which is filled with immature T cells and the medulla which is filled with mature T cells
What other cells inhabit the thymus?	Branched cortical and medullary epithelial cells, macrophages, and dendritic cells
What role do macrophages in the thymus play?	Removal of thymocytes that fail to mature properly
What role do bone marrow stromal cells provide in B cell development?	They release different cytokines which trigger B cell development and attachment
What part of the bone marrow do immature B cell inhabit?	The subendosteum
What are the two central or primary lymphoid tissues?	Thymus gland and bone marrow
What is extramedullary hemopoiesis	It the process by which the liver and spleen will attempt to produce blood cells if the bone marrow becomes too diseased
What are peripheral or secondary lymphoid tissues?	Lymph nodes, lymph, gut-associated lymphoid tissue, and spleen
What cell is the most prominent within the lymphoid follicle of a lymph node?	B cell
Where are T cells the most prominent within the lymph node?	Lymphoid paracotex

Physiology

What are the 3 types of granulocytes?	Neutrophils Basophils Eosinophils
What are the 3 types of agranulocytes?	Lymphocytes Monocytes Platelets
Where do thymic precursors come from?	Bone marrow
Which part of the thymus do immature T cells enter?	The subcapsular or outer cortex of the thymus
What is the first receptors thymocytes express?	CD2, which is a T cell specific adhesion molecule
As they move into the inner cortex what happens?	They interact with the branching network of epithelial cells and express both CD4 and CD8 receptors (called double-positive T cells)
What is positive selection?	It is a process in cortex where the CD4 and CD8 receptors are tested and only one is maintained on the single-positive T cell
Which type of MHC class do CD4 receptors interact with?	Type II
Which type of MHC class do CD8 receptors interact with?	Type I
What is negative selection?	That is the process by which a T cell is shown a self-peptide in the cortico-medullary junction. If their receptor binds too strongly, then they undergo apoptosis
Where does the final stage T cell develop occur?	In secondary lymphoid tissue
What triggers these naive T cells to divide and differentiate?	Interact with their receptor specific antigen
What do CD4+ T cells further mature into outside the thymus?	T helper 1 or 2 cells

What are B cells derived from?	Pluripotential hemtopoietic stem cells
What are the B cell develop stages called?	Early pro-B cell→ late pro-B cell→ pre-B cell→ immature B cell→ mature B cell
What do immature B cells express?	Only IgM
What can mature or naive B cells express	IgM or IgD
The final stage of B cell maturation occurs where?	Either in the bone marrow or in secondary lymphoid tissue
What is a plasma cell?	A mature B cell that secretes antibodies
What is a memory B cell?	A post-immune-response, differentiated, high-affinity, quick acting B cell, that enables a second encounter with an antigen to be faster and stronger

Biochemistry

Antibodies are made of what building blocks?	They are glycoproteins, composed of 4 polypeptides with with a carbohydrate attachment
What allows for antibodies to react to a plethora of antigens?	Different amino-acid sequences on the variable region allows diversity among antigen-binding specificity.
What role does Vitamin A play in the immune system?	Maintains mucosal and epithelial lining and secretions and proper B cell and T cell functions
What role does Vitamin E play in the immune system?	It is necessary to prevent membrane peroxidative damage in T cells, and to a lesser extent in B cells
What role does Vitamin C play in the immune system?	It increases neutrophil and monocyte chemotaxis and its antioxidant properties help maintain a defense against oxidative species
What role does Vitamin D play in the immune system?	It effects T cell proliferation and enhances cytokine production

What role does Zinc play in the immune system?	It enhances natural killer cell activity
What role does Selenium play in the immune system?	It affects glutathione peroxidase and phospholipid hydroperoxide, which help reduce arachidonic acid

Pathology

Bacteriology

What bacteria is associated with buboes?	*Yersinia pestis*
What distinguishing feature differentiates *Escherichia coli* from *Shigella* and *Salmonella* in vitro?	*Escherichia coli* ferments lactose, and the others do not.
What agar is used to help diagnose *Escherichia coli*?	MacConkey agar
Pink colonies on MacConkey agar indicates what?	Lactose fermentation
What are the other distinguishing features that can be useful for diagnosing *Escherichia coli*?	*Escherichia coli* is: indole positive, motile, methyl red (MR) positive, Voges-Proskauer (VP) negative, Citrate negative.
Which *Streptococcus* spp. are beta-hemolytic?	*Streptococcus pyogenes* (group A), *Streptococcus agalactiae* (group B)
Which *Streptococcus* spp. is alpha-hemolytic?	*Streptococcus pneumoniae*
What infection is caught from raw milk and is especially dangerous for pregnant women and newborns?	*Listeria monocytogenes*
What is the route of transmission of *Yersinia pestis*?	Rat carries fleas that harbor the bacteria and spread it to humans
Which of the following is not a lactose fermenter: *Proteus, Escherichia, Klebsiella, Enterobacter*?	*Proteus*

What species causes typhoid fever?	*Salmonella typhi*
What causes epidemic typhus?	*Rickettsia prowazekii*
What causes endemic typhus?	*Rickettsia typhi*
What are some of the symptoms of typhus?	Macular rash, high fever, severe myalgia and headache, arthralgias, signs of sepsis including hypotension
What organism causes rose colored spots on the abdomen, high fever and possible perforation of the abdomen?	*Salmonella typhi*
Salmonella cholerasuis = *S. enterica* causes what three diseases primarily?	Pneumonia, osteomyelitis and meningitis
What Gram positive cocci is catalase positive?	*Staphylococcus aureus*
What Gram positive cocci is catalase negative?	*Streptococcus*
What allows *Staphylococcus aureus* to resist penicillin?	Penicillinase which destroys penicillin.
The catalase test is diagnostic for what organism?	*Staphylococcus aureus*
What organism has hemolysis as a diagnostic feature?	*Steptococcus*
What are the two pigments secreted by *Pseudomonas aeruginosa* that can be helpful in diagnosis?	Pyocyanin Pyoverdin
What is a distinguishing feature of pyocyanin?	It can turn the pus in an infected wound blue
What color will pyoverdin fluoresce under UV light?	Yellow-green
What organism is responsible for scarlet fever?	*Streptococcus pyogenes*

What immunological sequelae can follow a *Streptococcus pyogenes* infection?	Rheumatic fever or glomerulonephritis
In what type of *Streptococcus* infection is the capsule pathogenic?	*Streptococcus pneumoniae*
What STD grows on a Thayer-Martin agar in CO_2?	*Neisseria gonorrhea*
Which STD is oxidase positive?	*Neisseria gonorrhoea*
What disease has a slow spreading circular lesion called erythema migrans?	Lyme disease
What disease can you get from improperly home-canned products?	Botulism, due to *Clostridium botulinum*
People who handle livestock are susceptible to what kind of infection?	*Bacillus anthracis*
What are the most serious complications of diphtheria?	Respiratory paralysis and death
What infection results in a gray pseudomembrane in the throat?	*Corynebacterium diphtheriae*
What is a common cause of purulent otitis media in children, as well as causing meningitis and pneumonia?	*Haemophilus influenzae* B
What organism grows around *Staphylococcus aureus* on agar plate?	*Haemophilus influenzae*
What is so special about *Mycoplasma* species morphology?	They have no cell wall and therefore are resistant to penicillin.
What organism is cultured in armadillos?	*Mycobacterium leprae*
What general kind of organism causes Lyme disease and syphilis?	Spirochetes
Yaws is caused by what organism?	*Treponema pallidum pertenue*
What are some of the lab tests for syphilis?	VDRL, FTA-ABS, RPR, MTA-TP, and darkfield microscopy
What organism causes glue ear?	*Haemophilus influenzae* B

What organism has a blue-green pigment and is associated with skin and especially burn infections?	*Pseudomonas aeruginosa*
What is the vector for Lyme disease?	Various ticks, most notably in the USA the deer tick, *Ixodes scapularis*
Lyme disease closely parallels what other disease in its primary, secondary and tertiary symptoms?	Syphilis
What species of organisms are transmitted by arthropods?	*Rickettsiae*, arboviruses
Rickettsiae typhi affects which type of cells?	Endothelial cells
What is the vector for *Rickettsia prowazekii*?	The louse
What is the vector for *Rickettsia typhi*?	The flea
What is the only rickettsial disease with no vector, and what organism causes it?	Q fever caused by *Coxiella burnetti*
What is the organism responsible for Rocky mountain fever?	*Rickettsia rickettsii*
How is Rocky mountain spotted fever transmitted?	Wood tick (*Dermacentor andersoni*) or dog tick (*Dermacentor variabilis*) bites
What disease is associated with standing water e.g. in air conditioning systems, and what organism causes it?	Legionnaire's disease, *Legionella pneumophila*
What disease is associted with birds?	*Chlamydia psittaci*
Parrot fever is the common name for what disease, caused by what organism?	Psittacosis caused by *Chlamydia psittaci*

Mycology

What is the common name for the clinical presentation of *Coccidiodes immitis* or *Coccidiodes posadasii* infection?	San Joaquin Valley fever, formally coccidioidomycosis
From what do fungi derive their energy, and how is this different from plants?	From organic chemicals, primarily saccharides, unlike photosynthesis in most plants.
Residence in what region of North America is a risk for contracting coccidioidomycosis?	Southwestern US, Northwestern México, and Central America
Residence in what region of North America is a risk for contracting histoplasmosis?	Northeastern US in Ohio and Mississippi river valleys
Residence in what region of North America is a risk for contracting Blastomycosis?	States bordering the Mississippi and Ohio rivers and those states and provinces bordering the Great Lakes and St. Lawrence River
What is the most common clinical presentation for someone infected with *Coccidiodes immitis*?	Flu-like illness (fever, chest pains, cough, and weight loss)
Who is most likely to developed serious complications or meningial involvement if infected with *Coccidiodes immitis*?	Immunodeficient individuals, pregnant women, Those with blood group B, and those of African and Filipino decent
What are the acute symptoms of a Blastomycosis infection?	looks like a bacterial pneumonia (myalgia, arthralgia, chills, fever, and cough) potentially with bone, skin, or male gentiourinary involvement
What are the acute symptoms of a Histoplasmosis infection?	Mild flu-like illness (fever, headache, malaise, pleuritic chest pain, and nonproductive cough)
Which primary fungal infection has primary lung involvement with secondary mucosal lesions?	Paracoccidioidomycosis cause by *Paracoccidioides brasiliensis*
How do yeast reproduce?	Asexual budding
How do molds reproduce?	Spores, can be formed by meiosis (sexually) or mitosis (asexually)

What is the tubular branching network of a mold technically called?	Mycelium or colony
What is the name of the tubular branches of a mold?	Hyphae and Pseudohyphae
What are the two types of Hyphae?	Coenocytic (hollow and multinucleate) Septate (Septate contain groups of cells surrounded by a tubular cell wall and divided by a porous Septum which allows for the sharing of cytoplasm and organelles)
How do pseudohyphae and hyphae differ?	Pseudohyphae do not share cytoplasm or organelles between cells
Do yeast contain hyphae?	No, they are unicellular
How can a mold be differentiated from a yeast under the microscope, and can an organism switch between the two forms?	Mold has hyphae, yeast are single rounded cells; and organisms can switch between them or at least go between a yeast form and a pseudohyphae-forming form.
What substance predominates in the fungal cell wall?	Chitin
What steroidal substances predominates in the fungal plasma membrane?	Ergosterol
What medically important fungus is an obligate anaerobe?	None! (unlike bacteria)
What primary fungal pathogen is associated with bat and bird feces?	*Histoplasma capsulatum*
What opportunistic fungal pathogen is associated with bird feces?	*Cryptococcus neoformans*
What large capsulated yeast is commonly found in pigeon droppings?	*Cryptococcus neoformans*
Dermatophytes survive by obtaining nutrients from what?	Keratin
How is Tinea diagnosed?	KOH wet mount, Wood's light or Fungal culture

How is Candida diagnosed?	Gram stain, KOH wet mount, vaginal pH, and skin biopsy
What opportunistic yeast most commonly overgrows in immunocompromised patients?	*Candida albicans*
How do you differentiate between a cutaneous Candida and Tinea infection?	Candida affects skin folds and the scrotum and has satellite lesions versus Tinea corporis doesn't affect skin folds and Tinea crusis doesn't affect the scrotum
What organisms cause jock itch (tinea cruris)?	*Trichophyton rubrum, Trichophyton mentagrophytes Epidermophyton floccosum*
What organism causes tinea barbae?	*Trichophyton verrucosum*
Chronic histoplasmosis can clinically resemble what other infectious disease?	Tuberculosis
What is the purpose of adding potassium hydroxide (KOH) to wet mounts?	Dissolves human skin while leaving yeast cells intact.
What is the purpose of using India Ink?	It is used primary to detect *Cryptococcus spps.*

Virology

What lymphoid cell is most affected by Epstein-Barr virus (EBV)?	B lymphocytes
What two diseases are associated with EBV?	Infectious mononucleosis Chronic fatigue syndrome
What infection is defined by the appearance of multinucleated giant cells with intranuclear inclusions inside organ tissues?	Cytomegalovirus (CMV)
How is EBV distinguished from CMV?	Monospot test for EBV (heterophile antibodies) or by detecting anti-CMV IgM in a blood sample
What is the gold standard test for CMV?	Tissue culture

What is the characteristic finding found in tissue staining for CMV?	"Owl's eyes" bodies, otherwise known as basophilic intranuclear inclusion body surrounded by a clear halo.
Human herpes virus-6 is associated with what exanthum?	Roseola infantum
Roseola infantum is associated with what characteristic macular rash? What other virus can cause this?	The slapped cheek rash; parvovirus B19 (a.k.a. erythrovirus B19)
What are the four pathogenic viruses in the Paramyxovirus family?	Measles Mumps Respiratory syncytial virus (RSV) Parainfluenza viruses.
What virus is associated with German measles?	Rubella
What is the incubation period of rubella?	14–21 days
Rubella infection is associated with what outcome if contracted by pregnant women?	Congential malformation in the heart, the eyes, and/or brain in the fetus in the first trimester.
How is rubella spread?	Respiratory droplets
What is the name of the virus that causes measles?	Rubeola
What skin presentation is virtually diagnostic for measles? Where does it appear? What does it look like?	Koplik's spots on the buccal mucosa; bright red lesions with a white center.
What is the incubation period for measles?	7–14 days.
What are the prodromal signs and symptoms of measles?	Fever Cough Rhinitis Conjunctivitis

What symptoms typically accompany the rash of measles?	1. Photophobia 2. Cough 3. Conjunctivitis 4. Pruritus 5. Leukopenia 6. Leukocytosis
What progressive, usually fatal brain disorder is associated with measles?	Subacute sclerosing panencephalitis
Where are the most common sites for common warts?	Fingers Hands Elbows
How is mumps transmitted?	Respiratory droplets
What is the incubation period of mumps?	14–24 days
Mumps is initially associated with the swelling of what tissue?	Parotid glands
What condition in postpubertal males is associated with mumps?	Bilateral orchitis
The common cold is caused most commonly by which viruses?	Rhinovirus, coronavirus, RSV, adenovirus, parainfluenza, metapneumovirus
Epidemics of influenza are associated with what strain of the virus? Why?	Influenza A, related to its large number of hosts (compared to influenza B which infects only humans and seals).
Pandemics of influenza are associated with what changes in the virus?	Antigenic shift, major changes in RNA
How is Coxsackie virus spread?	Fecal-oral route
What diseases are associated with coxsackie virus?	Myocarditis/pericarditis Meningitis/encephalitis Respiratory infections Hand-foot-mouth disease
The rhabdovirus is associated with what disease?	Rabies
The formation of what in the CNS is a hallmark sign of rabies?	Negri bodies

What is the incubation period of rabies?	30–50 days
Alpha and flavi viruses are spread by what vector?	*Aedes aegypti* mosquitoes
What three diseases are associated with alpha and flavi viruses?	Yellow fever Dengue fever Viral encephalitis e.g. St. Louis and West Nile virus
Human immunodeficiency virus (HIV) has tropism for what types of cells in the body?	CD4+ T-helper lymphocytes
What are the most common routes of HIV transmission?	Contact with blood Sexual intercourse with exchange of bodily fluids Placentally During birth Via breast milk
How is a preliminary diagnosis of HIV made?	Via a positive ELISA test
If a patient gets a positive ELISA test what do you follow up with?	A confirmatory Western Blot test
What does it mean that HIV is a retrovirus?	RNA virus that uses reverse transcriptase in a host cell to generate DNA which is then incorporated into the host genome via integrase so that the virus can then be replicated by the host cell.
What is envelope of an enveloped virus made of?	Host plasma membrane lipids and glycoproteins and some viral glycoproteins.
What are the most important enveloped viruses in medicine?	Herpes and pox viruses Dengue and yellow fever Rubella Viral encephalitis HBV and HDV Influenza, RSV, metapneumonavirus, parainfluenza Rabies Retroviruses

Parasitology

What organism causes amoebic dysentery? Can this disease manifest as bloody diarrhea?	*Entamoeba histolytica;* yes
What organism causes beaver fever? Can this disease manifest as bloody diarrhea?	*Giardia lamblia;* no
What parasite has as its definitive host the cat?	*Toxoplasma gondii*
Pneumocystis carinii overgrows in what kind of patient?	Immunocompromised
Who is most at risk for serious complications if infected by *Toxoplama gondii?*	The fetus of a pregnant woman
Which parasite interferes with fat absorption?	*Giardia lamblia*
What is the vector for African sleeping sickness?	Tsetse fly
What organism causes African sleeping sickness?	*Trypanosoma brucei*
What is the common name for *Ascaris lumbricoides?*	Human roundworm
What is the common name for *Necator americanus?*	Hookworm
What parasite causes spoon nails, anemia and stunted growth?	Hookworm
What parasite can be contracted from pork or bear meat?	*Trichinella spiralis*
How is filariasis transmitted?	Mosquito
What causes elephantiasis?	The parasitic worms *Wuchereria bancrofti, Brugia malayi,* and *B. timori;* non-filarial disease in Eastern Africa is thought due to chronic contact with irritant soils.
Schistosoma spp. are associated with what reservoir?	Snails

Taenia spp are associated with which animals?	Pigs, cows
What kind of parasite is *Taenia spp*?	Beef or pork tapeworm
Diphyllobothrium latum is what kind of parasite?	Fish tapeworm
What kind of parasite is a schistosome?	A blood fluke
Does *Toxoplasma gondii* form cysts?	Yes

Immune Reactions

The role of B lymphocytes is categorized as what kind of immunity?	Humoral
What is produced with humoral immunity?	Antibodies
The role of T lymphocytes is categorized as what kind of immunity?	Cell-mediated
What type of chemical activates components of the immune system ie. activates macrophages, PMNs etc.?	Lymphokines
Which white blood cell is the most numerous in the blood stream?	Neutrophil
What is the function of basophils?	They function in the inflammation response by releasing histamine and other chemicals that act on the blood vessels
Basophils become what in peripheral tissue?	Mast cells
What is the function of neutrophils?	They recognize foreign antigens and destroy them through phagocytosis
What is the function of eosinophils?	They release IgE and destroy parasitic organisms
Once maturing, where do eosinophils migrate to from bone marrow?	After 3-8 hours in the blood stream, they migrate to the skin, lungs, and GI tract
What is the function of monocytes/macrophages?	They engulf foreign antigens and cell debris and process antigen and present it.

Give examples of monocytes throughout the body.	Liver Kupffer cells, pulmonary alveolar macrophages, dendritic antigen-presenting cells, sinus lining cells of the spleen and lymph node, and free macrophages of the synovial, pleural, and peritoneal fluid.
What is the function of B lymphocytes?	They are independently able to identify foreign antigens and differentiate into antibody producing plasma and memory cells
What human cytokine stimulates B lymphocytes?	Interleukin-2
What is the role of T lymphocytes?	T helper cells induce B lymphocytes, T supressor cells recognize and kill virus infected cells
What is the function of natural killer cells?	Cells that bond to and lyse other cells especially those infected with virus
What on a cell's surface marks it as an antigen-presenting cell?	MHC class II expression
The four loci of the human leukocyte antigen (HLA) system have a strong influence on what physical states?	a. Human allotransplantation b. Transfusions in refractory patients c. Specific disease associations
What cells are classified as antigen-presenting dendritic cells?	Langerhans' cells in skin, dendritic reticulum cells of lymph nodes, follicular dendritic cells, interstitial dendritic cells, microglia of CNS
What is the principal immunoglobulin in exocrine secretions e.g. breast milk, respiratory and intestinal mucous, saliva and tears?	IgA
What immunoglobulin can move across the placenta thus becoming an important imuunoglobulin for newborns?	IgG
What is the main immunoglobulin in serum?	IgG

What immunoglobulin activates complement and is important in opsonization?	IgG
What immunoglobulin attaches to mast cells in the respiratory and intestinal tracts and plays an important role in allergic response?	IgE
What immunoglobulin is the first to form in response to an attack?	IgM
What immunoglobulin controls the A, B, O blood group antibody responses?	IgM
Antigens present on all nucleated cells in the body that identify a cell as self are called what?	HLA
What is a hapten?	A substance that normally does not act as an antigen
Complement is activated in what kind of immune reponse?	B-cell mediated immune response
What kind of proteins are involved in vasodilation, chemotaxis, opsonization of antigen, lysis of cells and blood clotting?	Complement
In the complement activation system what is the difference between the classic and alternative pathway?	The classic pathway is activated by C1's contact with antigen-antibody complexes and the alternative pathway is activated by C3's contact with various structures (e.g. bacterial polysaccharides, complex polysaccharides, or aggregated IgA). Both result in cleaving of C3 and the activation of complement.
Which complements are responsible for the release of histamine by mast cells?	C3a and C5a (known as anaphylatoxins)
Which complement is responsible for leukocyte activation, adhesion, and chemotaxis?	C5a

Which complements are responsible for the membrane attack complex?	C5b-C9
Which complement acts as an opsonin for phagocytes?	C3b
What is opsonization?	A coat is placed on cells so that they can be recognized
What role does interferon play?	They are released when invading organism is a virus. They inhibit production of virus in infected cells, prevent viral spread, enhance activity of macrophages, NK cells, cytotoxic T cells and inhibit growth of tumor cells.
Which interleukin permits cells of immune system to talk to one another and initiates response?	Interleukin-1
Which interleukin promotes cellular immunity ie. promote growth and activity of macrophages and B cells?	Interleukin-2
Which interleukins promote humoral immunity?	Interleukins-4, -5 and -10
Allergies are what type of hypersensitivity reaction?	Type I
How does the cell first respond to an antigen in a normal and an allergic Type I hypersensitivity reactions?	a. Normal: Bound B-cell goes to a T-cell to be activated with initial exposure to an antigen b. In allergies: the B-cell goes to a Type 2 T- helper cell, which releases IL-4 and causes the B-cell to produce IgE antibodies to the antigen

What happens during the second exposure to an antigen in an allergic Type I hypersensitivity reaction?	a. In the second exposure, the antigen binds to bound IgE, causing release of histamine and leukotriene granules from mast cells and basophils b. Degranulation causes vasodilation, vascular permeability, smooth muscle contraction and varying degrees of response from hives to anaphylactic shock
What occurs during anaphylactic shock?	Vascular permeability causes fluid accumulation in the lung, dropping blood pressure and triggering shock. Bronchioles are constricted.
What is a Type II hypersensitivity reaction?	A cytotoxic reaction from an antigen-antibody response, in which cytotoxic cells and complement are activated
What are two examples of a Type II hypersensitivity reaction?	Goodpasture's syndrome Pernicious anemia
What is a Type III hypersensitivity reaction?	Immune complexes are deposited in vessels or tissue, activating complement
What are three examples of Type III hypersensitivity reaction?	Polyarteritis nodosa Acute glomerulonephritis Serum sickness
A cell mediated or delayed reaction mediated by the interaction of antigen with T lymphocytes and subsequent release of lymphokines is an example of what type of hypersensitivity reaction?	Type IV
What are examples of Type IV hypersensitivity reactions?	Contact dermatitis Thyroiditis Allograft rejection
IgE is formed in what type of hypersensitivity reaction?	Type I
The reaction of antigen and antibody in extracellular fluid spaces is what type of hypersensitivity reaction?	Type III

What Type III hypersensitivity reactions occur in systemic lupus erythematosis (SLE)?	a. Vasculitis: damage to blood vessels, causing the characteristic butterfly rash and damaging heart valves b. Glomerulonephritis: damage to kidney glomeruli c. Arthritis: damage to synovial joints
Tuberculosis is an example of what type of hypersensitivity reaction?	Type IV
Loss of normal tolerance by the immune system of "self" antigens on the surface of the body's cells with destruction of normal tissue with autoantibodies is defined as what?	Autoimmunity
During an infection or inflammatory state otherwise latent anti-self lymphocytes become activated by foreign pathogens resembling self, they then produce an immune reaction to the foreign substance and the self is called what?	Moleular mimcry or cross-reaction autoimmunity
What is an example of molecular mimcry?	An initial steptococcal infection can be followed by rheumatic heart disease because antibodies to the streptococcal M protein cross-react with cardiac glycosides

Clinical Immunology

Hla-B27 is associated with what condition?	Ankylosing spondylitis
Hla-DR4 is associated with what conditions?	Rheumatoid arthritis, juvenile diabetes
What are the three types of anti-receptor antibodies?	a. Anti-receptor antibodies that activate the receptor b. Anti-receptor antibodies that block the receptor c. Anti-receptor antibodies that bind without receptor interference
What is a classic example of blockage by anti-receptor antibodies?	Myasthenia gravis, in which antibodies are formed against the acetylcholine receptor, interfering with normal muscle function

What is an example of a condition caused by activating anti-receptor antibodies?	Graves' disease, in which the TSH receptor is activated without regard to amount of thyroid hormone
How do autoimmune diseases occur?	Loss of immune system tolerance for self-antigen or cross-reaction
What autoimmune disease affects the epithelial desmosomes?	Pempgius
Patients with Sjögren's disease have a 40 times greater risk of developing what condition?	Lymphoma
What occurs with progressive systemic scleroderma?	The epidermis of the skin atrophies and the dermis thickens and fibrosis develops at the corners of the mouth
What symptoms occur in the CREST form of scleroderma?	a. Calcification b. Raynaud's phenomenon c. Esophageal dysphagia d. Sclerodactyly e. Telangiectasia
How do polymyositis and dermatomyositis typically develop?	Both develop immune-mediated muscle inflammation and vascular damage. In polymyositis, the immune system acts against unrecognized muscle antigens. In dermatomyositis, endomysial vessels and the microvasculature of the dermis are damaged by complement
Rheumatoid arthritis is what type of hypersensitivity reaction?	Type III hypersensitivity reaction
Agammaglobulinemia is an immune system defect causing an absence or low level of the gamma fraction of serum globulin, predisposing individuals to what types of conditions?	Frequent infections of the mucous membranes, sinuses, eyes, ears, airways, GI tract, and lungs
Patients with common variable immunodeficiency (CVID) have impaired antibody responses and a marked reduction in the serum levels of what immunoglobulins?	IgG and IgA, and more than half have reduced IgM

What is the most common of the immunodeficiency diseases?	IgA deficiency
What types of conditions are associated with IgA deficiency?	a. Recurrent ear infections, sinusitis, pneumonia b. Allergies c. Asthma: selective IgA deficiency d. Food allergies e. Certain autoimmune diseases, including rheumatoid arthritis and SLE
What is DiGeorge's syndrome?	A developmental issue results in thymic hypoplasia and therefor a T-cell deficiency
What is X-linked agammaglobulinemia?	A genetic error results in B cells not being able to develop beyond the pre-B cell stage which means a lack of circulating antibodies
What types of infections would a person with X-linked agammaglobulinemia not be able to clear?	Extracellular bacterial infections
What are the characteristics of severe combined immunodeficiency (SCID)?	a. Thymus atrophy b. Lack of delayed hypersensitivity c. Susceptibility to bacterial, viral, fungal and protozoal infections and infections from live vaccines
What are the early symptoms of HIV infection?	An acute illness similar to mononucleosis and persistent generalized lymphadenopathy
What are organisms are known to cause opportunistic infections in patients with AIDS?	Pneumocystis carinii Cytomegalovirus Candida Cryptosporidium Toxoplasma
What is a fast-growing opportunistic disease in AIDS patients?	Kaposi's sarcoma

The analysis and identification of DNA, RNA, and proteins via a blotting tool are called what?

DNA identification is called a Southern blot

RNA identification is called a Northern blot

Protein identification is called a Western blot

Integumentary System

Embryology

What germ layer forms the connective tissue?	Mesoderm
What germ layer forms the epidermis?	Ectoderm
From what do the dermis and hypodermis arise?	Mesoderm
What germ layer forms the retina of the eye?	Ectoderm
What is the lanugo?	A downy coat of delicate hairs that cover a 5-6 mo old fetus

Anatomy

What are the two distinct layers of the skin?	Epidermis and dermis
Which layer is vascularized?	The dermis
What is the hypodermis also known as?	The superficial fascia or subcutaneous tissue below the skin
What is the role of the hypodermis?	To connect the skin to the underlying tissue and stores fat
What cells inhabit the epidermis?	Keratinocytes, melanocytes, Merkel cells, and Langerhans' cells
What role do keratinocytes play?	They produce keratin, which hardens the epidermis

What role do melanocytes play?	Synthesize a melanin pigment that helps protect the epidermis from UV damage
What role do Merkel cells play?	They are sensory receptors for touch
What role do Langerhans' cells play?	They are epidermal macrophages
What is the connective tissue sheet called that supports the eyelids?	The tarsal plates
What are the glands called that are embedded in the tarsal plates?	Tarsal or Meibomian glands
What muscle operates the opening of the superior eyelid?	Levator palpebrae superioris
What is the role of the conjunctiva?	To produce lubricating mucus that prevents drying out of the eyes
What is the white of the eye called?	Sclera
What is contained within the lacrimal fluid?	Mucus, antibodies, and lysozymes (bacteria destroying enzyme
What type of photoreceptor is found in the fovea?	Just cones no rods

Physiology

What do you call the type of cells that comprise the epidermis?	Keratinizd stratified squamous epithelium
What makes up sweat?	99% water with salts, vitamin C, antibodies, a microbe-killing peptide, and lactic acid

Cellular Physiology

What are the 3 types of epithelium?	Simple Pseudostratified Stratified
What are the 3 shapes of epithelial cells?	Squamous, cuboidal, columnar
Which organelle regulates and initiates all cellular activity?	Nucleus

Which organelle is the site of synthesis of ribosomal RNA?	Nucleolus
Which organelle is the site of energy production?	Mitochondrion
Which organelle is the storage area for calcium?	Mitochondrion
Which ER had ribosomes?	Rough ER
In which organelle does protein synthesis take place?	Rough ER
In which organelle does CHO, steroid and fat synthesis take place?	Smooth ER
Protein containing vesicles leave the rough ER destined for which organelle?	The Golgi apparatus
Which organelle modifies proteins by adding CHO to make glycoproteins?	Golgi apparatus
What is the machinery of intracellular digestion of cellular debris called?	Lysosomes
What are the names of particles that contain the machinery for translation of genetic code into protein?	Ribosomes
Where do peroxisomes originate?	From the smooth ER
What role do Glycolipids play in the cell membrane?	They are responsible for intercellular communications (usually comprised of sphingolipids.)
What structures help distribute cell organelles, transport macromolecules within the cell and help shape the cell during differentiation?	Microtubules
What is the name for microfilaments in muscle?	Myofilaments
What organelle has a high concentration of oxidative enzymes?	Peroxisomes

INTEGUMENTARY

What structure gives membrane its integrity?	Phospholipids
What are the three most common phospholipids in the cell's membrane?	Phosphatidylcholine, Phosphatidylserine, and Phosphatidylethanolamine
What does an increase in cholesterol do to the membrane?	It decreases the fluidity of the membrane making it hard and less permeable
Active transport requires what?	ATP
Facilitated transport requires what?	Specific membrane transport protein
How does a substance move in passive transport?	Via simple diffusion down its concentration gradient
Transportation in and out of a cell is termed what?	Endocytosis and exocytosis
What are the 3 types of endocytosis?	Phagocytosis, pinocytosis, and receptor mediated endocytosis
How does water move in osmosis?	Water moves from an area of low solute concentration to an area of high solute concentration.
How do RBCs react to an isotonic solution?	No change in size
How do RBCs react to a hypertonic solution?	They shrink
How do RBCs react to a hypotonic solution?	They swell
Large particles moving into a cell by invagination of the cell membrane is a process of what?	Phagocytosis
List 4 support cells?	Fibroblasts, Chondrocyte, Osteoblast, Myofibroblast, Adipocyte
True or False: Myofibroblasts help with retraction of fibrocollagenous scars?	True, they activate during the repair phase of tissue damage. They produce collagen and contract in order to reduce the physical size of the wound

What are 7 epithelial cell junctions?	Occluding or Tight junction Anchoring junction Adherent junction Desmosomes Hemidesmosome Junctional complex Gap or Communication Junctions
What makes up the extracellular matrix and what produces it?	Support cells produce the extracellular matrix which is mainly composed of fibrillar proteins and glycosaminoglycans
What are the 2 types of adipocytes?	Unilocular (e.g. white fat) and multilocular (e.g. brown fat)
Which adipocyte is more prominent in infants?	Multilocular, which contain numerous mitochondria and lipid vacuoles which allow for greater heat generation through fat breakdown

Teperature Regulation

Which organs contribute to core temperature?	Brain Heart Kidney and liver
What are 3 ways to measure temperature?	Rectally Orally Axillary
Which of the 3 methods of measuring temperature is more accurate?	Rectal
What are the 4 ways of losing body heat?	Radiation Evaporation Conduction Convection
What condition makes people especially vulnerable to hypothermia?	Windy conditions
Since we gain heat from radiation and conduction from objects around us, what is the only real means of losing heat?	Evaporation

What 2 methods does the body use to lose heat?	Vasodilation especially of cutaneous vascular beds and sweating
What 2 things are strongly inhibited when the body is trying to lose heat?	↓ Shivering ↓ Thermogenesis
What hormone is closely related to increasing Basal metabolic rate?	Thyroxine secretion from the thyroid gland
What role do epi and norepi play in heat production?	They uncouple oxidative phosphorylation which will ↑ cellular metabolism to produce heat and not ATP
What are three methods of heat production other than ↑ cellular metabolism?	Shivering Vasoconstriction Piloerection
What causes an increase in the thyroxine output?	Cooling of the preoptic area of hypothalmus →↑TRH →↑TSH →↑ thyroxine output
Where is the primary centre for shivering located?	In the posterior hypothalmus
What substances increase the set point of the hypothalmus?	Pyrogens
What causes the release of pyrogens?	Bacteria Degenerating tissues of the body WBCs in viral infections
What eicosanoid causes the fever increasing mechanism to "go off"?	Prostaglandin E1
What is the purpose of increasing the set point?	To provide an unhealthy environment for bacteria and viruses to live in

Biochemistry

What amino acid is the basis for melanin?	Tyrosine
What affect does carotene intake have on the skin?	It is a yellow-orange pigment found in plants that can accumulate in the stratum corneum
What vitamin is formed from the effects of sunlight on cholesterol in the skin?	Vitamin D

What nutritional deficiencies are associated with optic neuropathy?	Vitamin B12, thiamine, and folate
What vitamin is needed to produce retinol?	Vitamin A
Retinol is needed for what?	It is needed to bind with opsin to form rhodospin, which allows for vision in dim lights.

Pathology

Basic Pathology
Cellular Adaptation and Injury

What is it called when cells increase in size?	Hypertrophy
What are the 2 ways a cell undergoes hypertrophy?	In response to increased hormones In response to increased functional demand
What is hyperplasia?	A condition whereby the number of actual cells increase
What are the 3 ways hyperplasia develops?	In response to functional changes In response to persistent cell injury Increased hormones
What is it called when a cell shrinks in size?	Atrophy
What are some of the reasons for atrophy?	Cells shrink in size in response to: Persistent injury or pressure Decreased workload Loss of innervation Lack of blood supply Inadequent nutrition Loss of endocrine stimulation
Which type of muscle can undergo hyperplasia, hypertrophy, and atrophy?	Smooth Muscle
What is it called when one type of tissue converts into another type?	Metaplasia
What is a common cause of metaplasia?	Persistent injury
What is a loss of blood flow called?	Ischemia

What is a lack of blood flow to a tissue called?	Hypoxia
What is one of the most common causes of cell injury and degeneration?	Lack of oxygen
What are three ways that reduced ATP production from low oxygen in the tissues can cause tissue and cell damage?	a. Increase in anaerobic respiration (glycolysis) leading to an increase in lactic acid and a decrease in pH. b. Failure of ATP-dependent sodium potassium pump that increases the osmolarity of the cell and causes cloudy swelling of the cell, endoplasmic reticulum, and mitochondria. c. Failure of ATP-dependent calcium pump, which allows an increase in intracellular calcium.
What is necrosis?	The degradation that happens to cellular tissue after cell death, usually from irreversible cell injury.
What is the most common type of necrosis?	Coagulative necrosis
What do you call the necrosis that is marked by destruction of tissue by lysosomal enzymes?	Liquefactive necrosis
What type of necrosis is commonly seen with tuberculosis granulomas, which is marked by a soft-cheese like transformation of the tissue?	Caseous necrosis
What type of necrosis is most often associated with the lower limbs and ischemia?	Gangrenous necrosis
What type of necrosis is a complication of pancreatitis?	Enzymatic fat necrosis
What other type of tissue is affected by enzymatic fat necrosis?	Breast tissue
What is amyloidosis?	The inappropriate deposition of protein into tissue

What do you call the brown granules representing lipid-containing residues of lysosomal digestion?	Lipofuscin
What type of pigmentation is caused by the oxidation products of tyrosine in intracellular organelles in epidermal cells?	Melanin
What is programmed cell death called?	Apoptosis
True or False: Apoptosis can be triggered intrinsically or extrinsically?	True, extracellular signals can be from nitric acid or toxins and intraceullar signals can come from a lack of growth factors
What pathway does intrinsic apoptosis use?	Intrinsic apoptosis signals result in mitochondrial permeability with the release of death inducing proteins into the cytoplasm
What pathway does extrinsic apoptosis use?	Extrinsic apoptosis signals result in the initation of death receptors in the plasma membrane
What are death receptors in the plasma membrane?	Death receptors are comprised of members of the TNF receptor family, which have an intracellular domain involving protein-protein interactions which initiates the apoptotic cascade.
What is the name for the intracellular domain for protein-protein interactions that when activated initiates the apoptotic signal intracellularly?	The death domain
What do the extrinsic and intrinsic apoptotic pathways share in common?	They both initiate the caspase enzymes which activate

Inflammation

Acute inflammation occurs within what period of time?	Short duration, less than 72 hours
Which leukocyte dominates within the acutely inflamed tissue in the first the first 6-24 hours?	Neutrophil, they usually undergo apoptosis within 24-28hrs after exiting the blood stream.
Acute inflammation involves what cellular changes?	Neutrophil infiltration Swelling Edema
Chronic inflammation occurs after what period of time?	After 48–72 hours
Chronic inflammation involves what types of inflammatory cells and cellular changes?	Macrophages Lymphocytes Plasma cells Fibroblasts New blood vessels Tumor necrosis factor (TNF)
What are common causes of chronic inflammation?	Acute inflammation Viral infections Certain autoimmune diseases Parasites Malignant tumor
What is chemotaxsis?	It the process by which a leukocyte follows a chemical gradient that directs it from its extravascular site to the injury site
Name the 4 steps by which leukocytes move from the vascular lumen into the extravascular space during acute inflammation?	Margination, rolling, adhesion and transmigration
What is margination?	Larger white blood cells are pushed along the lumen wall whereas the smaller cells (i.e. red blood cells) move faster along the center of the lumen. This enables leukocytes to have elongated contact with the lining epithelial cells.

What is rolling?	As leukocytes move along the endothelial surface they transiently stick due to sugary receptors called selectin on both the leukocyte and endothelium.
What is adhesion?	When a leukocyte remains fixated to the endothelial surface. This firm adhesion is due to integrins on the leukocyte's surface and ICAM-1 and VCAM-1 on the endothelial surface. Integrins only bind to ICMA-1 and VCAM-1 when activated by chemotactic agents (TNF and IL-1) during inflammation.
What is transmigration?	Through the help of PECAM-1 on the endothelium and the leukocyte's surface, the leukocyte is able to squeeze between intercellular junctions and reach tissue
Cell injury causes an influx of calcium that does what?	Breaks down phospholipids and releases arachidonic acid
Why are steroids anti-inflammatory?	Steroids inhibit phospholipase
What inhibits the cyclo-oxygenase pathway?	Aspirin and non-steroidal anti-inflammatory agents
What chemical mediators cause vasodilation following cell injury?	Prostaglandins, especially PGI_2 (prostacylcin)
What chemical mediators cause vasoconstriction?	Thromboxanes
What is the main leukotriene for adhesion and chemotaxis in inflammation?	LTB_4
What occurs when Factor XII comes into contact with collagen or activated platelets?	Production of bradykinin and activation of the clotting, fibrinolytic and complement cascades.
What causes the degranulation of histamine-containing vesicles?	Trauma, cold, immune reactions
When are the effects of histamine felt during an inflammatory reaction?	During the first 30 min

Which cells release histamine in inflammation?	Basophils, platelets, and mast cells (only mast cells contain pre-formed histamine).
What is another name for platelets and what are they differentiated from?	They are known as thrombocytes and they come from megakaryocytes.
Which cells release serotonin in inflammation?	Platelets. It is usually released during platelet aggregation.
What does nitric oxide promote?	Vascular permeability
What does nitric oxide inhibit?	Platelet aggregation
What amino acid is nitric acid formed from?	Arginine
What vascular changes may occur in the body following massive tissue injury or serious infection?	Levels of TNF-alpha rise may rise and cause systemic vasodilation and shock
What are two examples of long-term damage that results from inflammatory complications?	Hepatic cirrhosis and emphysema
When is tissue regeneration possible?	When the basement membrane is intact and when tissues are made up of cells capable of mitosis
What does the process of fibrosis involve?	a. Inflammation b. Liquefaction and clearing of dead cells and debris c. Formation of granulation tissue d. New capillaries proliferate Fibroblasts generate collagen to create scar tissue

General Carcinogenesis

What is a papilloma?	Benign tumor of epithelial cells projecting outward either micro- or macroscopically
What is a polyp?	Benign tumor projecting macroscopically into a lumen
What premalignant situation exists if dysplastic or neoplastic cells have not breached the basement membrane?	Carcinoma in situ

What are the four most common types of malignant tumors?	a. Sarcoma: malignant tumor of mesenchymal tissue b. Carcinoma: malignant tumor of epithelial tissue c. Adenocarcinoma: carcinoma with a glandular pattern d. Squamous cell carcinoma: carcinoma arising from stratified squamous epithelium
Which cells are most susceptible to becoming neoplastic?	Epithelial cells
What is the "two-hit hypothesis" of cancer development?	It takes more than one genetic mutation for a cell to become cancerous
What are some of the major sources of mutagenic and carcinogenic compounds?	a. Tobacco products b. Food c. Water d. Chemical exposures e. Radiation exposures f. Drugs
What must occur for a cell to go through full neoplastic transformation and become a malignant tumor?	Multiple genetic abnormalities
What two types of genes are involved in carcinogenesis?	a. Oncogenes b. Tumor suppressor genes
What is an proto-oncogene called after it mutates?	Oncogene
When tumor suppressor genes mutate, what may potentially occur in the cell?	The cell may potentially divide forever
As tumors enlarge, what do they promote around them?	a. Neo-angiogenesis b. Lymphangiogenesis
How do cancer cells evade detection by the immune system?	They develop mutations altering cell surface markers and secrete immunosuppressive compounds

How do neoplastic cells facilitate local invasion into adjacent tissues?	a. Loss of contact inhibition b. Secretion of enzymes, such as matrix metalloproteases, that dissolve connective tissue
What are two cancers that tend to metastasize by venous drainage and settle in specific sites in the body?	a. Prostate cancer: pelvis and lumbar spine b. Lung cancer: brain
What are two areas of the body with fine capillary beds that are common sites of metastasis in the body?	Lung and liver
How long does it take a single malignant cell to become clinically detectible?	30 population doublings
What is the primary reason tumors grow in size?	Cells produced are immortal and accumulate
What are some examples of complications and systemic effects caused by malignant tumors?	a. Immune suppression b. Metastasis c. Micrometastasis d. Indirect malignancy e. Cachexia f. Hemorrhage g. Paraneoplastic syndromes h. Pathological fractures i. Hypercoagulability j. Resistance to therapy
What is one of the most common reasons people actually die from cancer?	Many tumors secrete compounds that induce cachexia, causing wasting
What are some examples of tumors that are curable by surgery alone if caught early?	a. Malignant melanoma b. Breast cancer
When a tumor is being graded, what is an important factor to be assessed?	Degree of differentiation of cells, with less differentiated cells termed anaplastic cells
How is the mitotic index used when assessing malignant tumors?	It is used to identify cells with rapid mitosis and determine grade and prognosis

How does receptor analysis help determine prognosis with various cancers, such as breast cancer?

Receptor analysis helps identify those cancers susceptible to hormonal controls and guides therapeutic choices, such as the use of hormonal therapies, e.g., **tamoxifen** use in estrogen-receptor positive patients with breast cancer

How are most malignant tumors staged?

Tumors are staged by determining:
T: size and extent of local invasion of tumor
N: lymph node involvement
M: whether there is distant metastasis

What are some tumor markers that are sometimes used for cancer screening, though most are too non-specific for general use?

a. Alpha Feto-Protein (AFP)— testicular cancer and heptocellular cancer
b. Human Ghorionic Gonadotropin (HCG)— testicular cancer
c. Prostate-specific antigen (PSA)— prostate cancer
d. Carbohydrate Antigen 125 (CA-125)— ovarian and other cancers
e. Carcinoembryonic Antigen (CEA)— colorectal cancer
f. Carbohydrate Antigen 19–9 CA19–9— pancreatic cancer

Genetics

What are the three most common types of genetic mutations?

a. Point mutations: single base pair alteration in DNA that causes a single amino acid change in a protein
b. Deletion and frame shift: reading frame change in DNA replication caused by single base pair removal
c. Trinucleotide repeats: base pair triplicates repeat, leading to proteins with many repeating amino acids

What type of mutation causes sickle cell anemia?

Point mutation

What is a karyotype?	A karyotype demonstrates the chromosomal characteristics of a cell or cell line. In a karyotype, metaphase chromosomes from a single cell nucleus are arranged in an array of pairs in descending order of size and position of the centromeres
What are the 3 types of inheritance patterns?	a. Autosomal dominant b. Autosomal recessive c. X-linked
Familial hypercholesterolemia is an example of what type of inheritance pattern?	Autosomal dominant, in which there is partial or complete absence of LDL cholesterol receptors
What are some examples of autosomal recessive disorders?	a. Phenylketonuria (PKU), a defect of phenylalanine hydroxylase leading to an inability to catabolize Phe b. Lysosomal storage diseases, such as Tay-Sachs disease c. Glycogen storage diseases
What are some examples of conditions with multifactorial/polygenic causes?	a. Atherosclerosis b. Diabetes mellitus type II c. Hypertension d. Allergies e. Cancer f. Cleft lip and palate

Dermatology & ophthalmology

What are the two major organisms that cause impetigo?	*Staphylococcus aureus* *Streptococcus pyogenes*(group A, beta-hemolytic)
What type of toxin is responsible for the scalded skin syndrome of *Staphylococcus aureus* infection?	Exfoliatin
What organism is associated with hot tubs and can cause folliculitis?	*Pseudomonas aeruginosa*
What causes gas gangrene?	*Clostridium perfringens*

What organism causes most boils, carbuncles, and impetigo?	*Staphylococcus aureus*
What is the medical name for ringworm?	Tinea corporis
What are the different types of Tinea?	Tinea cruris (groin) Tinea pedis (feet) Tinea corporis (face, trunk, limbs) Tinea capitis (scalp) Tinea barbae (beard) Tinea manuum (hands)
How are herpes simplex viruses (HSV) mainly transmitted?	Salivary or vesicle fluid contact, can be infected by asymptomatic shedding
What can cause a relapse of HSV?	Stress, hormonal fluctuations, environmental changes, illness, dietary factors
What are common locations for HSV-1 outbreaks?	Face, lips
Is the initial lesion of herpes painful or painless?	Painful
What are the most common tests for diagnosing HSV infection?	Cell culture, ELISA or PCR testing
Downey cells or atypical lymphocytes are seen in infection with what virus?	EBV
What is the virus that causes chickenpox (varicella)?	Varicella-zoster virus (VZV)
Painful vesicles that emerge along a dermatome are associated with what disease?	Shingles (herpes zoster)
What is the incubation period for chickenpox?	14–21 days
What type of rash is associated with chickenpox?	Pruritic (itchy), papulovesicular rash
Warts on the feet are called what?	Plantar warts

What is urticaria?	Flattened, fluid-filled, pruritic vesicles appearing in response to a type I hypersensitivity reaction
How do all eczemas generally present?	Redness, unclear margins, scaling, pruritis, and lichenification
Atopic dermatitis is frequently associated with what conditions?	Asthma and hay fever
Seborrheic dermatitis is generally associated with what type of inflammatory reaction?	Inflammatory response toPityrosporum yeasts and their breakdown products
What causes contact dermatitis?	Acute exposure to an antigenic substance
What is erythema multiforme?	Sudden inflammatory reaction causing symmetric erythematous, edematous, or bullous lesions of the skin and mucous membranes, possibly due to drugs or infectious agents
Where does psoriasis most commonly occur?	Extensor surfaces of elbows and knees
What are the four Ps of lichen planus?	Pruritic Polygonal-shaped Pink papules Purple papules
What are the two types of pemphigous?	a. Pemphigus vulgaris: most severe form, with intraepidermal bullae that begin in the mouth and spread b. Bullous pemphigoid: less severe form, with itchy bullae
What are seborrheic keratoses?	Benign neoplasm affected older individuals that have a pasted on appearance
What is the underlying infection in verrucae (warts)?	Infection with human papilloma virus (HPV)
Actinic keratoses have a propensity to develop into what skin condition?	Squamous cell carcinoma
How does basal cell carcinoma present?	As a pearly papule on sun-exposed skin

If a nevi (mole) is changing shape or becoming irregular or ill defined, what might be necessary?	Biopsy to assess for melanoma
What occurs during the development of melanoma?	a. Initial growth is radial and without metastasis, so is most easily cured in this stage b. Subsequent growth is vertical through the tissues and metastasis more common, with a worse prognosis
An infection in the tarsal glands resulting in a cyst is called what?	Chalazion
Glaucoma is caused by what?	A blockage of the canal of Schlemm resulting in a build-up of aqueous humor and thus the intraocular pressure
What is the medical term for being nearsighted	Myopia, which is due to a long eyeball
Vitamin A decificency can lead to what?	Rod degeneration which causes Night Blindness
Congenital weakness of external eye muscle can cause what?	Strabismus
What occular pathology is associated with auto-immune conditions?	Uveitis
What are the key notes of Hypertensive Retinopathy?	a. Narrowing and irregularity of retinal arteries b. Arteriovenous nicking c. Blot retinal hemorrhages d. Microaneurysms e. Cotton-wool spots
What are the key features of Diabetic Retinopathy?	a. Microaneurysms b. Retinal Hemorrhages c. Retinal lipid exudates d. Cotton-wool spots e. Capillary nonperfusion f. Macular edema g. Neovascularization

Musculoskeletal System

Embryology

What germ layer forms smooth muscle coat?	Mesoderm
What germ layer forms smooth muscle?	Mesoderm
What germ layer forms the skeleton?	Mesoderm
What germ layer forms the striated muscle?	Mesoderm
What are the 4 supports cells (fibroblasts, chondrocytes, oestoblasts, and myofibroblasts) derived from?	Mesenchyme

Anatomy

Arthrology

What is an example of a syndesmosis joint?	Distal tibiofibular joint (tibiofibular syndesmosis)
What is an example of a plane/gliding/arthrodial joint?	Acromioclavicular Calcaneocuboidal Carpometacarpal (except jt. of thumb) Intercarpals Proximal tibiofibular
What is an example of a hinge joint?	Elbow Talocrural (ankle) Interphalangeal Mandible Knee
What is an example of a condylar joint?	Metacarpophalangeal Atlanto-occipital

What is an example of a ball and socket joint?	Hip Shoulder
What is an example of an ellipsoidal joint?	Wrist
What is an example of a pivot/trochoid joint?	Distal radioulnar Atlas/axis
What is an example of a saddle joint?	Carpometacarpal joint of thumb (between trapezium and MC1)
What is an example of a symphysis joint?	Pubic symphysis
What type of joint forms the fibrous union between the radius and ulna?	Syndesmosis joint
What type of joint is a cranial suture?	Synarthroid
Fibrous joints that are either immovable or barely movable are classified as what type of joint?	Synarthrosis
What type of joint is united by hyaline cartilage or fibrocartilage?	Cartilaginous
What type of joint is united by an articular capsule and allows free motion in at least one axis?	Synovial or diarthrodial joint

Axial Skeleton

What are the four main sutures in the skull?	The Coronal, Sagittal, Squamous, and Lambdoid
What suture separates the parietal bone and the temporal bones from the occipital bone?	Lambdoid suture
What suture separates the parietal bones superiorly?	Sagittal suture
What suture separates the parietal bone from the temporal bone laterally?	Squamous suture
What suture separates the frontal bone from parietal bones?	Coronal suture

What forms the bregma landmark?	The intersection of the coronal and sagittal sutures
Which bones are considered pneumatized bones (i.e. contain sinuses)?	Frontal bone Temporal bone Sphenoid bone Ethmoid bone
What is the easily palpable, external occipital protuberance on the medial plane between the inferior and superior nuchal lines of the occiput called?	The inion
What bone forms the posterior part of the nasal septum?	Vomer
What bones make up the nasal aperture?	Nasal Maxilla Frontal
What makes up the septum?	Vomer Septal cartillage Perpendicular plate of the ethmoid bone
The inion is associated with which bone?	Occiput
Which bone of the skull has the styloid process?	The temporal bone
What bones make up the hard palate?	Palatine bone Maxilla
What prominence on the mandible forms the prominence of the chin?	Mental protuberance
What are the articular surfaces involved in the TMJ?	Head of condylar process of the mandible articulates with the mandibular fossa and articular tubercle of the temporal bone
What ligament limits post. movement of TMJ?	Lateral Temporomandibular ligament
What passes through the optic canal?	Optic nerve (CN II) and Opthalmic artery
What structures pass through the superior orbital fissure?	Opthalmic veins, sympathetic fibers, CN III, CN IV, CN V_I (ophthalmic nerve), and CN VI

What passes through the mandibular foramen?	Inferior alveolar nerve a banch of CN V_3 (mandibular nerve) and the Inferior alveolar artery and vein
What exits through the stylomastoid foramen?	The facial nerve (CN VII) and stylomastoid artery
What passes through the mental foramen?	The mental artery and mental nerve a branch of CN V_3 (mandibular nerve)
What passes through the foramen rotundum?	The maxillary nerve (CN V_2)
What passes through the foramen ovale?	The mandibular nerve (CN V_3) and accessory meningeal artery
What passes through the supraorbital foramen?	The supraorbital nerve a branch of CN V_1 (opthalmic nerve)
What passes through the infraorbital foramen?	The infraorbital nerve a branch of CN V_2 (maxillary nerve)
What structures pass through the foramen lacerum?	Internal carotid artery and accompanying sympathetic and venous plexuses
What bones make up the auditory ossicles?	Malleus Incus Stapes
What U-shaped bone lies at the level of C3 vertebrae?	Hyoid bone
What makes up the primary curves of the spine?	Thoracic curve Pelvic (Sacrum/coccyx) curve
What makes up secondary curves of spine?	Cervical curve Lumbar curve
What type of curve is the lordotic curve?	Secondary
What type of curve is the kyphotic curve?	Primary
Which are the true/movable vertebrae?	Cervicals Thoracics Lumbars

What are the false/fixed vertebrae?	Sacrum Coccyx
What makes up a typical vertebra?	Vertebral body 2 pedicles 2 laminae 4 articular processes 2 Transverse processes 1 spinous process
Which of the cervical vertebrae are atypical?	C1, C2, C7
Which of the thoracic vertebrae are atypical?	1, 10, 11, and 12
Which of the lumbar vertebrae are atypical?	L5
Where is the 1st intervertebral disc found?	Between C2 and C3
Where does head flexion take place?	Between Atlas and occiput
Where does head rotation take place?	Between Atlas and axis
What penetrates the atlanto-occipital membrane?	suboccipital nerve Vertebral artery
What ligament spans the inside of the vertebral foramen on the posterior side?	Ligamentum flavum
What ligament prevents full rotation of the head?	Alar ligament
What ligament holds the dens in ventral position?	Cruciform
What ligament is found on the dorsal surface of the inside of the vertebral foramen?	Ligamentum flavum
What ligaments join tips of vertebral spines?	Supraspinous ligs.
What ligaments span between vertebral spines?	Interspinous ligaments

What forms the boundary for the intervertebral foramen?	Superior and inferior vertebral notch
What is contained within the intervertebral foramen?	Spinal nerve Intervertebral artery and vein Intervertebral lymphatic vessels Adipose tissue Peripheral nerve roots and meningeal sleeves
What vessels and nerves pass through the intervertebral foramen?	Spinal nerve Intervertebral artery and vein Intervertebral lymphatic vessels
What passes through the transverse foramina of the cervical vertebrae?	The vertebral artery and vein
The vertebral artery does NOT pass through the transverse foramina of which cervical vertebra?	C7
Which CNs pass through the jugular foramen?	CN IX, X. XI
How many articulations are there between a typical rib and vertebrae?	3: head of rib articulates with 2 vertebral bodies; tubercle on neck of rib articulates with 1 TVP
What ligament is involved with the head of the rib connecting with the vertebral body?	The radiate ligament
How many true ribs are there?	7
What constitutes a true rib?	The first 7 ribs that are attached to the sternum by their own costal cartilage
Which ribs are called vertebrochondral ribs?	Ribs 8, 9 and 10
Which ribs are typical ribs?	Ribs 3 to 9
What constitutes a typical rib?	They contain a head, a tubercle and a shaft (a.k.a. a body)
Which is the most curved, broadest and shortest rib?	Rib 1

What attaches to the scalene tubercle on the 1st rib?	The anterior scalene muscle
What passes through the groves anterior and posterior to the scalene tubercle on the 1st rib?	Anterior grove = The subclavian vein Posterior grove = the subclavian artery and lower brachial plexus
Which ribs have only one facet each on their heads?	Ribs 1, 10, 11 and 12
What structure gives elasticity to the thoracic wall?	Costal cartilage
True or False: There is a cervical rib?	True, it occurs in 0.5% of the population and arises from the 7th cervical vertebra's transverse process.

Appendicular Skeleton

What is the name of the structure produced by the meeting of the manubrium and the body of the sternum?	The angle of Louis, aka the sternal angle
What part of the sternum lies at the level of T3 and T4?	Manubrium
What portion of the sternum lies at the level of T10?	Xyphoid
Give the landmarks for when the trachea begins and ends?	It begins at 6th cervical vertebra and extends to the level of the sternal angle
What joint forms the junction of the xiphoid and the sternum?	Xiphisternal joint
What are the 3 angles of the scapula?	Inferior Superior Lateral
What are the 4 fossa on the scapula?	Supraspinatus fossa Infraspinatus fossa Subscapular fossa Glenoid cavity
What are the 2 tubercles on the scapula that are superior and inferior of the glenoid cavity?	Supraglenoid tubercle Infraglenoid tubercle

What lateral continuation of the spine of the scapula articulates with the clavicle?	Acromion
What 2 ligaments make up the capsular ligaments of the shoulder?	Coracohumeral ligament Glenohumeral ligament
What is the chief bracing ligament of the acromial end of the clavicle?	Coracoclavicular ligament
What ligament prevents superior displacement of the humeral head?	Coracoacromial
Superior displacement of the humerus will likely damage what ligament?	The acromioclavicular ligament
What provides the main stability for the glenohumeral joint?	Rotator cuff tendons
What muscles make up the rotator cuff?	Supraspinatus Infraspinatus Teres minor Subscapularis
What ligament of the elbow does the ulnar nerve pass through?	The ulnar collateral ligament
What ligament holds the head of the radius in position in the proximal radioulnar joint?	Annular ligament
The radius articulates with which 3 carpal bones to form the radiocarpal joint?	Scaphoid Lunate Triquetral
What ligament attaches to the ulnar styloid process and the radius to provide support for the distal radioulnar joint and preventing the ulna from touching the wrist joint?	Articular disc
Which bone of the forearm takes on the weight bearing function in the wrist?	The radius
Which fingers have sesamoid bones?	1,2,5
Which ligament prevents hyperextension of the knee?	Anterior cruciate ligament

Which ligament prevents posterior displacement of the femur on the tibia?	Anterior cruciate ligament
Which ligament prevents anterior displacement of the femur on the tibia?	Posterior cruciate ligament
Which of the collateral ligaments of the knee is extracapsular?	Lateral (fibular) collateral ligament
What ligament attaches to the tibial tuberosity?	The patellar ligament
Ligament of the head of the femur is also known as what?	Ligamentum teres
Which of the collateral ligaments is attached to which of the menisci?	The medial meniscus is attached to the tibial/medial collateral ligament
Which ligament of the knee limit side to side movement?	Collateral ligaments
Which bursa of the knee facilitates full flexion and extension?	Suprapatellar
Which bursa of the knee is associated with housemaid's knee and permits movement of skin over the patella during leg movement?	Subcutaneous prepatellar bursa
Which bursa is associated with clergyman's knee?	Subcutaneous infrapatellar bursa
What bones are joined by the spring ligament?	Calcaneus (sustentaculum tali) navicular (medial side of foot)
What ligament prevents the talus from wedging bones apart?	The spring ligament
The ankle/talocrural joint is supported by what ligament on the medial side?	The deltoid ligament
What ligaments support the lateral aspect of the talocrural/ankle joint?	Anterior and posterior talofiular ligaments Calcaneofibular ligament
During what movement is the ankle joint most unstable?	During plantar flexion (moving foot away from the body!)

Which ligaments are most likely to be injured with forced inversion (turning sole of foot medially)?	Anterior and posterior talofibular ligament Calcaneofibular ligament
Which of the talofibular ligaments is least likely to tear?	Posterior talofibular ligament
Inversion and eversion of the ankle occurs at which joints?	Talocalcaneonavicular joint Talocalcaneal joint
What ligament supports the longitudinal arch?	Spring ligament
Which toe has sesamoid bones?	Big toe

Myology

What does the orbicularis oculi muscle do?	Closes eye
What muscle elevates, adducts and rotates eyeball medially?	Superior rectus
What muscle depresses, adducts and rotates eyeball medially?	Inferior rectus
What muscle abducts the eyeball?	Lateral rectus
What muscle adducts the eyeball?	Medial rectus
What muscle abducts, depresses and rotates eyeball medially?	Superior oblique
What muscle abducts, elevates and rotates eyeball laterally?	Inferior oblique
What muscle elevates the upper eyelid?	Levator palpebrae
What eye muscles are innervated by CN III?	Superior rectus Inferior rectus Medial rectus Inferior oblique Levator palpebrae
What eye muscles are innervated by CN IV?	Superior oblique
What muscles are innervated by CN VI?	Lateral rectus

What 2 muscles open the mouth?	Digastric Lateral pterygoid
What 3 muscles close the mouth?	Temporalis Masseter Medial pterygoid
What muscles make up the pillars of the fauces?	Palatoglossal Palatopharyngeal
What are the muscles of swallowing?	The constrictor group
What nerves innervate swallowing?	CN IX (Glossopharyngeal) and CN X (Vagus)
What do the intrinsic muscles of the tongue do?	Alter shape of tongue
What muscle sticks tongue out?	Genioglossus
What muscle pulls tongue back into mouth?	Styloglossus
What muscle elevates tongue?	Palatoglossus
What muscle depresses tongue?	Hyoglossus
What does palatopharyngeus do?	It raises the tongue to the palate.
Which of the muscles that moves the tongue is innervated by CNX (Vagus)?	Palatoglossus
What nerve innervates most of the motor actions of the tongue?	CN XII (Hypoglossal nerve)
What innervates touch of the ant. 2/3 of the tongue?	Lingual nerve, a branch of the mandibular division (V_3) of the trigeminal nerve (CN V)
What innervates taste of ant. 2/3 of tongue?	CN VII (facial nerve), chordatympani branch
What innervates touch and taste for the post. 1/3 of tongue?	CN IX (glossopharangeal)
What do tensor palati and levator palati do?	Raise and tauten the soft palate

CN VII, the facial nerve, has partial innervation of which of the muscles of mastication?	Digastric
What is the main nerve for muscles of mastication?	CN V$_3$ (mandibular nerve)
What does palatopharyngeus muscle do?	Depresses the soft palate
Which muscle elevates the larynx?	Stylopharyngeus
What does the salpingopharyngeus muscle do?	Opens the auditory tube
What are the functions of the scm?	Rotation, flexion and lateral bending of the head/neck
What muscles make up the supra hyoid group?	Stylohyoid Digastric Myolohyoid Geniohyoid
What muscles make up the infrahyoid group?	Sternohyoid Sternothyroid Thyrohyoid Omohyoid
What group of muscles depresses the larynx and hyoid bone?	Infrahyoids
What group of muscles raises larynx and hyoid bone?	Suprahyoids
Which muscles close the epiglottis?	Aryepiglottis Thyroepiglottis Oblique arytenoid
Which muscles are involved in vocalization?	Posterior cricoarytenoid Lateral cricoarytenoid Arytenoid
Which muscle lengthens and thus causes a lower pitch?	Cricothyroid
What muscles shorten and thus cause a higher pitch?	Thyroarytenoid and vocalis

What nerve innervates motor to the cricothyroid muscle?	Superior laryngeal nerve
What nerve innervates to the remaining laryngeal muscles?	Recurrent laryngeal nerve
What muscle of the neck connects the cervical vertebrae?	Longus colli
Which of the prevertebral muscles attach atlas to occiput?	Rectus capitis anterior Rectus capitis lateralis
What suboccipital muscles attach atlas to occiput?	Rectus capitis posterior minor Superior oblique
What suboccipital muscles attach axis to the occiput?	Rectus capitis posterior major
What suboccipital muscle attaches atlas to axis?	Inferior oblique
What muscles make erector spinae group?	Spinalis Longissimus Iliocostalis
Which of the erector spinae is closest to the spine?	Spinalis
What muscles make up the transversospinalis group?	Semispinalis Multifidus Rotatores
What muscles flex the neck?	Longus colli Longus capitis Rectus capitis anterior SCM
What muscles laterally flex the neck?	Rectus capitis lateralis SCM
The brachial plexus emerges from which muscles?	Anterior and medial scalene
What muscles raise the ribs causing inhalation?	External intercostals
What muscles help with exhalation?	Internal intercostals

What nerve innervates the diaphragm?	Phrenic nerve
What forms the anterior border of the axilla?	Pectoralis major and minor
What forms the posterior border of the axilla?	Subscapularis Teres major Lattisumus dorsi
What forms the medial wall of the axilla?	Serratus anterior
What 3 muscles flex the humerus?	Pectoralis major Deltoid Coracobrachialis
What 3 muscles extend the humerus?	Lattisimus dorsi Teres major Deltoid
What 2 muscles abduct the humerus?	Middle deltoid Supraspinatus
What 3 muscles adduct the humerus?	Pec major Lattisimus dorsi Teres major
What 3 muscles laterally rotate the humerus?	Infraspinatus Teres minor Posterior deltoid
What 5 muscles medially rotate the humerus?	Pec major Lattisimus dorsi Teres major Subscapularis Anterior deltoid
What 4 muscles flex the forearm?	Biceps Brachialis Brachioradialis Pronator teres
What 2 muscles extend the forearm?	Triceps Anconeus
What 2 muscles pronate the forearm?	Pronator teres Pronator quadratus

What 2 muscles supinate the forearm?	Supinator Biceps
What action does serratus anterior produce?	Protraction and rotation of scapula
What nerve passes over the anatomical snuff box?	The superficial radial nerve
What makes up the Anatomical snuffbox?	Scaphoid, Abductor policis longus, Extensor policis longus, Radial artery (remember with the acronym SABER)
What innervates the intrinsic muscles of the hand?	Ulnar nerve
What are the muscles that give us a power grip?	Forearm flexors
What nerve innervates the power grip muscles?	Median nerve
Wrist drop will occur with damage to which nerve?	Radial nerve (nerve to all the wrist extensors)
Damage to what nerve causes claw hand?	Ulnar nerve damage results in a loss of innervation to the interossei and lumbricals.
Which fingers are most affected in a claw hand deformity?	The 4th and 5th
Damage to what nerve causes Papal benediction?	Median nerve
What provides the roof of the carpal tunnel?	Flexor retinaculum
Do you get any loss of cutaneous sensation with carpal tunnel syndrome?	No because the ulnar nerve and the cutaneous branch of the median nerve do not pass through the carpal tunnel
What makes up the border of the tunnel of guyon?	Pisiform and hook of hamate
What muscle elevates the testes?	Cremaster

MUSCULOSKELETAL

The inguinal ligament is the lower free edge of what muscle?	External oblique
What muscles of the abdomen attach to the linea alba?	External oblique Internal oblique Transversus abdominis
Which abdominal muscle flexes the spine?	Rectus abdominis
The lowest tendinous fibers of transversus abdominis and internal oblique that attaches to the pubic crest and pectineal line is known as what?	Conjoint tendon
What weakens to form a direct hernia?	Conjoint tendon
What happens in an indirect hernia?	Protrusion of the intestine through the inguinal canal
What muscle raises the pelvic floor, supports pelvic viscera and controls defecation via elevation of the anal canal?	Levator ani
What attaches to the pubic bone?	Adductor group Pectineus (Pectineal line) Gracilis
What attaches to the iscial tuberosity?	Hamstrings
What attaches to the ASIS?	Sartorius Rectus femoris TFL
What forms the borders of the femoral triangle?	Sartorius Adductor longus Inguinal ligament
What forms the pes anserina?	Gracilis Sartorius Semitendinosus
What attaches to the greater trochanter?	Piriformis Obturator internus Gamellus superior Gamellus inferior Gluteus Maximus, medius, minimus

What muscles flex the knee?	Hamstrings Gastrocnemius
What muscles extent the knee?	Quadraceps
What laterally rotates knee?	Biceps femoris
What medially rotates the knee?	Semimembrinosus Semitendinosus
What attaches to the lesser trochanter?	Iliopsoas
What attaches to the tibial tuberosity?	Rectus femoris
What are the nine muscles that attach to the fibula?	Extensor hallucis longus Extensor digitorum longus Peroneus tertius Peroneus longus Peroneus brevis Soleus Flexor hallucis longus Tibialis posterior Biceps femoris
What 3 muscles dorsiflex the foot? What is the innervation?	Tibialis Anterior Extensor digitorum longus Extensor hallucis longus Peronius tertius Innervated by the deep peroneal nerve
What 2 muscles invert the foot?	Tibialis anterior: Deep peroneal nerve Tibialis posterior: Tibial nerve
What 3 muscles evert the foot?	Peroneus tertius: deep peroneal nerve Peroneus longus: superficial peroneal nerve Peroneus brevis: superficial peroneal nerve
What 5 muscles plantarflex the foot? What is the innervation?	Gastrocnemius Soleus Tibialis posterior Flexor digitorum longus Flexor hallucis longus Innervated by the tibial nerve

What dorsiflexes the toes? What is the innervation?	Extensor digitorum brevis Extensor hallucis brevis Extensor hallucis longus Innervated by the deep peroneal nerve
What passes posterior to the lateral malleolus?	Peroneus longus tendon Peroneus brevis tendon
What passes posterior to the medial malleolus?	Tibial artery, vein and nerve Tibialis posterior Flexor digitorum longus tendon Flexor hallucis longus tendon
What are the two branches of the tibial nerve?	Medial plantar nerve Lateral plantar nerve

Muscles and Actions of the Hip Movers

Flexors
Illiopsoas

Rectus femoris

Sartorius

1/2 of pectineus

Innervated by Femoral nerve

Extensors
Gluteus maximus

Biceps femoris

Semitendinosus

Semimembrinosus

Innervation by Sciatic nerve (exception: gluteus maximus is innervated by inferior gluteal nerve)

Abductors
Gluteus medius

Gluteus minimus

T.F.L

Innervation by Sup. gluteal nerve

Adductors

- Pectineus
- Gracilis
- Adductor group:
- Longus
- Magnus
- Brevis

Innervation by Obturator nerve

Medial rotators

- T.F.L.
- Gluteus minimus
- Gluteus medius
- Semi-membrinosus
- Semi-tendinosus

Lateral rotators

- Gluteus maximus
- Obturators
- Gamellis
- Quadriceps femoris
- Piriformis
- Iliopsoas
- Sartorius

Physiology

What are the 3 types of cartilage?	Hyaline Elastic Fibrous
What are the 4 types of bone cell?	Osteocytes Osteoclasts Osteoblasts Osteoprogenitor cells
What are the 3 types of muscle?	Skeletal Cardiac Smooth
What distinguishes hyaluronic acid from other glycosaminoglycans?	It has no sulphate bonds and is not protein-linked

Which glycosaminoglycan is the most abundant?	Chondroitin sulphate
What is the contractile unit of muscle?	The sarcomere
What is the name of the organelle in the muscle cell that is high in calcium?	Sarcoplasmic retinaculum
What is the neurotransmitter of the neuromuscular junction?	Acetylcholine
What substance fluxes through open gated channels when the action potential reaches the terminal bouton?	Calcium
The depolarization of the post synaptic membrane is known as what?	The End Plate Potential (EPP)
Why will the EPP always reach threshold every time?	Because it is suprathreshold
What stops the action of acetylcholine in the synaptic cleft?	Acetyl choline esterase
Adrenergic synapses use what neurotransmitter?	Norepinephrine
What are the 2 contractile proteins of muscle?	Actin and myosin
Which of the contractile proteins is found in the thin filament?	Actin
Which of the contractile proteins is found in the thick filament?	Myosin
What are the 2 regulatory proteins that are also found on the thin filament?	Troponin and tropomyosin
Which is the regulatory protein that has an inhibitory action on the formation of actin-myosin complex?	Tropomyosin
What substance causes the troponin-tropomyosin complex to fall away from the active site of the actin molecule?	Calcium

To which of the regulatory proteins does calcium bind?	Troponin
What substance is bound to the myosin head?	ATP
What to things do we need to get the muscle to relax?	a. Removal of calcium b. Formation of ATP on myosin head
Lifting and setting down contraction with muscle shortening and lengthening is known as what type of contraction?	Isotonic
Contraction with no external muscle shortening is what type of muscle contraction?	Isometric
The force-velocity curve describes what type of muscle contraction?	Isotonic (velocity gives sense of movement)
The length-tension curve describes what type of muscle contraction?	Isometric
Posture, heat generation, nerve nutrition of muscle and general circulation are all functions of what?	Muscle tone
What is it called when a series of action potentials reach a muscle such that it cannot relax and so force within a muscle is built to a maximum?	Summation of twitches
Accumulation of calcium in the cytoplasm is the mechanism for what?	Summation of twitches
What are the 3 muscle fiber types?	Fast oxidative glycolytic Slow oxidative Fast glycolytic
Marathon runners have more of what muscle fibers?	Slow oxidative
Sprinters have more of what type of muscle fibers?	Fast glycolytic
Where do you find smooth muscle in the body?	Hollow organs, blood vessels, lymphatics, in the skin to do piloerection and in the eye

What are the 2 different types of smooth muscle?	a. Multi unit b. Visceral-contracts as a single unit
Piloerection and the ciliary muscles of the eyes are examples of what type of smooth muscle?	Multi unit
Gap junctions are found in which type of smooth muscle?	Viscera
What is the cytoplasmic binding protein found in smooth muscle?	Calmodulin
What are 2 possible sources of calcium for smooth muscle contraction?	a. Mitochondrion b. Intracellular vesicles
How does relaxation of smooth muscle differ from relaxation of skeletal muscle?	It requires a light chain phosphatase enzyme to remove phosphate from myosin. In skeletal muscle relaxation is based on the reuptake of calcium and ATP formation on the myosin head.
What are the 2 types of action potentials in smooth muscle?	a. Spike potential b. Plateau potential
The gut, blood vessels experience what type of smooth muscle action potential?	Spike
The uterus and bladder experience what type of smooth muscle action potential?	Plateau potential
Smooth muscle contraction is regulated in what 2 ways?	a. Neurally i.e. via neurotransmitters b. Hormonally via blood borne agents (epi)and local tissue factors (O_2, CO_2, H^+)
What happens to smooth muscle when it is stretched?	It will often lead to a spike potential and contraction

Exercise Physiology

What happens to heart rate during an exercise bout?	It increases
What does the increase in heart rate during an exercise bout do to stroke volume?	Increases it
What happens to renal and splanchnic blood flow during an exercise bout?	They decrease
After the anaerobic threshold is reached during an exercise bout what causes an increase in ventilation?	↑ Lactic acid
What is the only metabolic hormone to be decreased in an exercise bout?	Insulin
What happens in skeletal muscle during an exercise bout?	1. ↑ in blood flow because vascular beds dilate and receive extra blood from renal and splanchnic beds 2. ↑ Metabolism up to 25X 3. ↑ Oxygen extraction
How does maximum heart rate get affected by training?	It remains unchanged
What happens to submax heart rate in a trained heart?	It decreases
What happens to the coronaries in a trained heart?	They increase in sizenot in number
How is stroke volume affected in a trained athlete?	It will ↑ because the heart is more efficient and better able to handle demands
How is oxygen consumption affected in a trained athlete?	It will ↓
What happens to mitochondrion content in a trained athletes skeletal muscle?	They ↑
What happens to capillary density in a trained athletes skeletal muscle?	It ↑
What happens to protein content of skeletal muscle with resistive training?	It will increase

What happens to lactate production in a trained athlete?	Less is produced for the same workload
Glucose and glycogen are spared due to the ↑ metabolism of what?	Fatty acids
What type of exercise will ↑ bone mass?	Weight bearing exercise
What kind of exercise will ↑ size and strength of ligaments and tendons?	Resistance training
How is insulin affected during rest and an exercise bout in a trained athlete?	**Rest:** lower insulin levels with higher sensitivity of receptors **Exercise bout:** higher insulin levels with lower sensitivity of receptors
What happens to epi, norepi, cortisol, glucagon and GH during and exercise bout in a trained athlete?	They experience a lower rise

Biochemistry

What role does creatine play in skeletal muscle metabolism?	It resynthesis ATP during strenuous exercise, buffers lactic acid, and stimulates protein synthesis and increasing muscle mass
What is creatine synthesized from?	The amino acids arginine, glycine, and methionine
What is the difference between glycogenolysis in skeletal muscle and the Liver?	Skeletal muscle lacks the enzyme needed to dephosphorylate glucose
How does that lack of enzyme effect the process?	Glucose is only partly oxidized into pyruvic or lactic acid
What happens to that lactic or pyruvic acid?	It reaches the blood and heads to the liver where it will be converted into glucose
What nutritional deficiencies are associated with myopathy?	Vitamin D and E

Pathology

What is Duchenne muscular dystrophy?	It is an X-linked disorder that is the most common and most severe muscular dystrophy. It is marked by wasting in the proximal muscles and extremities and compensatory hypertrophy of distal sites.
What causes myasthenia gravis?	It is an autoimmune disorder that develops from autoantibodies to acetylcholine receptors in the neuromuscular junctions.
What does pyogenic osteomyelitis most commonly affect?	The distal end of the femur and the proximal ends of the humerus and tibia.
Why is osteoporosis type I most commonly associated with post-menopausal women?	It is associated with estrogen deficiency, which occurs with menopause.
What causes an increase in hip fractures in people over 70 years of age?	Osteoporosis type II, which is caused by reduced calcium absorption.
Vitamin D deficiency is associated with what degenerative bone disease?	Osteomalacia
What are the most common types of skeletal tumors?	a. Osteoma: sessile tumor composed of well-formed bone b. Osteoid osteoma: small benign neoplasm, not malignant c. Osteosarcoma: most common primary malignant tumor of bone, usually occurring in males 10–20 years of age d. Chondrosarcoma: malignant cartilaginous tumor of men 30–60 years of age e. Ewing's sarcoma: anaplastic small-cell malignant tumor of long bones, ribs, pelvis, scapula, usually in boys under 15
What are some of the causes of infectious arthritis?	Gonorrhea, staph, strep, H. influenzae, rubella, mumps, hepatitis B, Lyme disease
What causes gouty arthritis?	Uric acid from the breakdown of purines is deposited as urate crystals in joints, particularly the metatarsophalangeal joint of the big toe.

What precipitates acute gout?	Large meal, alcohol
What joints are affected by rheumatoid arthritis?	a. Bilateral proximal interphalangeal (PIP) joints b. Metacarpophalangeal (MCP) joints c. Wrist joints
What types of deformities are associated with rheumatoid arthritis?	a. Haygarth's nodes on the PIPS b. Boutonniere or swan neck deformities on the fingers c. Ulnar deviation of the wrist d. Toe clawing
What is bamboo spine?	Fixation of the lumbar spine and sacroiliac joint in ankylosing spondylitis
What joints are affected in osteoarthritis?	Asymmetrical weight-bearing joints and distal interphalangeal (DIP) joints
What type of nodules form in osteoarthritis?	a. Heberden's nodes on the DIP joints b. Bouchard's nodes on the PIP joints
Osteochondrosis is a disease primarily affecting what age group?	Children

Neurological System

Embryology

What germ layer forms the central and peripheral nervous system?	Ectoderm
What happens after anteroposterior invagination of the neural placode?	The lateral ends fold to form the neural tube
What does the peripheral nervous system arise from?	The bifurcation of the neural crest and the closing of the neural tube
Once the neural tube has formed, what happens next?	Neuroepithelial cells proliferate resulting in neuroblasts
After proliferation what do the cells do?	They migrate to mature sites in order to establish synaptic connections and extend axons to target tissue
What are astrocytes and ependymal cells formed from?	Radial glial ells

Anatomy

Name the ventricles of the brain.	lateral ventricles, third ventricle, and fourth ventricle
How do the 2 lateral ventricles communicate with the third ventricle?	The interventricular foramina or foramn (aka the foramina of Monro)
What connects the 3rd and 4th ventricles?	Cerebral aqueduct
What divides the cerebral peduncle into an anterior part (the crus cerebri) and a posterior part (tegmentum)?	Substantia nigra

Where would you find the graciles tubercle?	Brain
How many cervical nerves are there?	8
How many coccygeal nerves are there?	1
At what level does spinal cord end?	L2
What are the nerve roots below L2 called?	The cauda equina
What does the brain stem consist of?	Medulla oblongata Pons Midbrain
What divides frontal and parital lobes?	Central sulcus
What separates frontal and temporal lobes?	Lateral sulcus
What separates the cingulate gyrus from the superior frontal gyrus?	The cingulate sulcus
What separates the cingulate gyrus from the corpus callosum?	Callosal sulcus
What does the cerebrum consist of?	The telencephalon and the diencephalon
What 4 structures make up the diencephalon?	Thalamus Hypothalamus Subthalamus Epithalamus
What parts make up the telencephalon?	cerebral cortex subcortical white matter Basal ganglia
What is the cerebellum comprised of?	2 lateral hemispheres divided by the vermis
What structure is connected to the hypothalamus by the infundibulum?	The pituitary gland is connected to the hypothalamus via the infundibulum and the infundibulum is considered part of the posterior lobe or the neurohypophysis
What part of the spinal cord contains the nerve bodies and unmyelinated fibers?	Gray matter

What part of the spinal cord contains somatic cell bodies and have motor functions?	Ventral or anterior horn
What part of the spinal cord contains visceral cell bodies and have visceral motor function?	Lateral horn
What part of the spinal cord contains the cell bodies of the neuron and have sensory functions?	Dorsal horn
What part of the spinal cord and brain contains an interconnecting nerve system which is made of the myelinated nerve fibers?	White matter
What are the four lobes of the brain?	Frontal Parital Temporal Occipital
What is the general function of the frontal lobe?	Motor function
What is the general function of the parietal lobe?	Somatosensory
What is the general function of the occipital lobe?	Vision
What is the general function of the temporal lobe?	Auditory
From superior to inferior what is the flow of CSF through the ventricles?	Lateral→Third→Fourth
From outside to inside what are the layers of the meninges?	Dura mater→Arachnoid mater→Pia mater
What kinds of nerve fibers are found in dorsal rami?	Sensory fibers carrying afferent information
What kinds of nerve fibers are found in ventral rami?	Motor fibers carrying efferent information
What are the spinal levels of the parasympathetic nervous system?	Brainstem—C1 S2,3,4

What are the spinal levels of the sympathetic nervous system?	T1-L2
Where is the primary somatic sensory cortex located?	Postcentral gyrus of the cerebral cortex
Where in the brain is the motor cortex located?	Precentral gyrus of the frontal lobe of both hemispheres
What portion of the brain is responsible for controlling the motor function of the muscles responsible for speech?	The Broca's area
What are the names of the three main ascending pathways?	Nonspecific ascending (Anterolateral) pathway Specific ascending (Lemniscal) pathway Spinocerebellar pathway
In what tract do pain and temperature travel?	In the lateral spinothalamic tract
In what tract does crude touch travel?	Anterior spinothalamic tract
In what tract do proprioception, tactile pressure, stereognosis, barognosis and 2 point discrimination?	In the gracillis and cuneatus fasiculi
which part of the ascending lemniscal pathway transmits information from upper limbs and upper trunk?	The fasciculus cuneatus
which part of the ascending lemniscal pathway transmits information from the lower limbs and inferior trunk?	The fasciculus gracilis
Which tract is concerned with subconscious perception ie. muscle and position sense pathway?	Spinocerebellar tract
Where do the anterior and lateral spinothalamic tract decussate?	At the level of the spinal cord at which they entered
Where do the gracillis and cuneate fasiculi decussate?	In the medulla
Where does the spinocerebellar pathway decussate?	It doesn't or it crosses over twice and cancels out the original decussation

Where does reticular formation take place?	The brain stem
Which portion of the brain stem controls autonomic function and houses the reflex centers for the respiratory, cardiac, and vasomotor system in addition to the reflex centers for vomiting, coughing, sneezing, and swallowing?	The medulla
What cranial nerves have their nuclei of origin in the midbrain?	CN III and IV
What cranial nerves have their nuclei of origin in the pons?	CN V,VI,VII
What cranial nerves have their nuclei of origin in the medulla?	CN VIII,IX,X,XI,XII
What Cranial nerve is responsible for the sense of smell?	Olfactory (CN I)
The Trigeminal Nerve is divided into what 3 nerves?	The Opthalmic Nerve (CN V1) The Maxillary Nerve (CN V2) The Mandibular Nerve (CN V3)
What nerves does the opthalmic nerve (CN V1) branch off into?	Frontal nerve (breaks into the Supraorbital and Supratrochlear nerve) Nasociliary nerve (branches into the Infratrochlear, Long ciliary, and Ethmoidal nerve, and Long root of the ciliary ganglion) Lacrimal nerve

What nerves does the maxillary nerve (CN V2) branch off into?	Middle Meningeal nerve Infraorbital nerve (which branches into the Superior Labial nerve branch) Zygomatic nerve (branches into the Zygomaticotemporal and Zygomaticofacial nerve) Superior Alveolar nerves (branches into the Posterior, Anterior, and Middle Superior Alveolar nerve) Inferior palpebral nerve Sphenopalatine (Pterygopalatine) ganglion (divides into the Nasopalatine branches, Palatine nerves (divides into the Greater and Lesser Palatine nerve), and the Pharyngeal nerves)
What nerves does the mandibular nerve (CN V3) branch off into?	Nervus spinosus Medial pterygoid nerve Buccal nerve Masseteric nerve Lateral pterygoid nerve Auriculotemporal nerve Lingual nerve Inferior Alveolar nerve otic ganglion
What nerve is responsible for lacrimal and salivary glands?	Facial nerve (CN VII)
what are the 5 main motor nerve branches of the Facial nerve?	Temporal, Zygomatic, Buccal, Mandibular, and Cervical
Which nerve's origin is in the pons and it supplies motor function to the lateral rectus muscle?	Abducens Nerve (CN VI)
Where are the superior cerebellar peduncles located?	Pons
Where is the substantia nigra located?	Midbrain
What part of the brain regulates the emotional state?	The limbic system
In what part of the brain do we consolidate short term memory into long term?	Hippocampus

In what part of brain do we find conditioned fear?	Amygdala
Where is dopamine released from?	Substantia nigra
What is released from raphe nucleus?	Serotonin
Where is norepinephrine released from in the brain?	Locus ceruleus
Which cranial nerves have parasympathetic action?	CN III, VII, IX, and X

Nerve and Nerve Root of Upper Extremity Muscles

MUSCLE	NERVE	ROOT	ACTION
Supraspinatus	Suprascapular	C4–C5	ARM: Abduction
Infraspinatus	Suprascapular	C5–C6	ARM: External rotation
Deltoid	Axillary	C5–C6	ARM: Flexion, extension, abduction, ext. rot.
Teres major	Lower subscap.	C5–C6	ARM: Extension, adduction, internal rotation
Teres minor	Axillary	C5–C6	ARM: External rotation
Subscapularis	Upper subscap.	C5–C6	ARM: Internal rotation
Pectoralis major	Lateral pectoral	C5–C7	ARM: Flexion, adduction, internal rotation
Latissiumus dorsi	Thoracodorsal	C6–C8	ARM: Extension, adduction, internal rotation
Coracobrachialis	Musculocutan.	C6–C7	ARM: Flexion, adduction
Trapezius	Spinal accessory	CN XI	SCAPULAR: Elevate, depress, retract, lat. rot.
Rhomboids	Dorsal scapular	C4–C5	SCAPULAR: Retract, elevate, medially rotate
Levator scapula	Dorsal scapular	C3–C5	SCAPULAR: Retract, elevate, medial rotation
Pectoralis minor	Medial pectoralis	C8–T1	SCAPULAR: Protract, dperess, medial rotation
Serratus anterior	Long thoracic	C5–C7	SCAPULAR: Protract, lateral rotation
Biceps	Musculocut.	C5–C6	ELBOW: Flexion, supination
Triceps	Radial	C7–C8	ELBOW: Extension
Brachialis	Musculocut.	C5–C6	ELBOW: Flexion
Brachioradialis	Radial	C5–C6	ELBOW: Flexion, supination
Anconeus	Radial	C7–C8	ELBOW: Extension
Supinator	Radial	C6	ELBOW: Supination
Pronator teres	Median	C6–C7	ELBOW: Flexion, pronation
Pronator quadratus	Median	C8–T1	ELBOW: Pronation
Flexor carpi radialis	Median	C6–C7	ELBOW: Flex, pronation. WRIST: Flex, radial dev.
Palmaris longus	Median	C7–C8	ELBOW: Flexion. WRIST: Flexion
Flexor carpi ulnaris	Ulnar	C8	WRIST: Flexion, ulnar deviation
Extensor carpi radialis longus and brevis	Radial	C6–C7	WRIST: Extension, radial deviation
Extensor carpi ulnaris	Radial	C7–C8	WRIST: Extension, ulnar deviation
Flexor digitorum profundis	Median	C8–T1	FINGERS: flexion (MCP, PIP, DIP)
Flexor digitorum superficialis	Median	C7–T1	FINGERS: Flexion (MCP, PIP)
Abductor policis brevis	Median	C8–T1	THUMB: Flexion, abduction, opposition
Lumbricals (fingers 1–2)	Median: 1–2	C8–T1	FINGERS: Flexion (MCP), extension (IPs)
Flexor policis longus and brevis	Median	C6–C7	THUMB: Flexion (Brevis: opposition)
Opponens policis	Median	C8	FINGER AND THUMB: Opposition
Opponens digiti minimi	Ulnar	C8–T1	FINGER AND THUMB: Opposition
Palmar interossei	Ulnar	C8–T1	FINGERS: Adduction, Flex (MCP), extend (IPs)
Dorsal interossei	Ulnar	C8–T1	FINGERS: Abduction, Flex (MCP), extend (IPs)
Lumbricals (fingers 4–5)	Ulnar	C8–T1	FINGERS: Flexion (MCP), extension (IPs)
Adductor policis	Ulnar	C6–C8	THUMB: Adduction, opposition
Extensor digitorum	Radial	C7–C8	FINGERS: Extension (MCP, PIP, DIP)
Extensor digitorum minimi	Radial	C7–C8	FINGERS: Extension (MCP, PIP, DIP)
Extensor digitorum indices	Radial	C7–C8	INDEX FINGER: Extension
Extensor policis longus and brevis	Radial	C7–C8	THUMB: Extension
Abductor policis longus	Radial	C7–C8	THUMB: Abduction, extension

Nerves of Muscles of the Forearm

Radial nerve

Muscles

1. Two extensors of the elbow

    Triceps

    Anconeus

2. One flexor of the elbow

    Brachioradialis

3. All extensors of wrist and fingers within forearm

    Extensor carpi radialis longus

    Extensor carpi radialis brevis

    Extensor carpi ulnaris

    Extensor digitorum

    Extensor digiti mini

    Extensor idicis

4. Extensors and long abductors of thumb

    Abductor policis longus

    Extensor pollicis brevis

    Extensor pollicis longus

5. One supinator of the forearm

    Supinator

Important locations: Travels over snuff box

Median nerve

Muscles

1. Two Pronators

    Pronator teres

    Pronator quadratus

2. One wrist flexor:

    Palmaris longus

3. Most flexors of the wrist and fingers within forearm:

    Flexor carpi radialis

    Flexor digitorum superficialis

    Flexor digitorum profundus (index and middle finger)

    Flexor pollicis longus

Important locations:

    Cubital fossa

    Through the carpal tunnel

Ulnar nerve
Muscles
1. Two flexors of the wrist and fingers
     Flexor carpi ulnaris
     Flexor digitorum profundus (little and ring finger)
Important locations:
     Posterior to medial epicondyle of humerus ("funny bone")
     Through the tunnel of guyon (space between pisiform and hook of hamate)

Nerves of Muscles of the Wrist and Hand

Ulnar Nerve
Muscles
1. Flex, abduct and oppose little finger
     Hypothenar group
2. One Adductor of thumb
     Adductor pollicis
3. Finger adductors
     Palmar interossei (PADs)
4. Finger abductors
     Dorsal interossei (DABs)
5. Flex MCP joint & Extend IP joint
     Ring and little finger lumbricals

Median Nerve
Muscles
1. Flex, abduct and oppose thumb
     Thenar group
2. Flex MCP joint & Extend IP joint
     Index and Middle Lumbricals

Radial Nerve
No innervation to muscles of wrist and arm

Cutaneous Innervation

Musculocutaneous nerve
Skin of anterior aspect of the upper arm and forearm

Median nerve

Skin of the anterior aspect of palm and anterior thumb, index, middle and 1/2 of ring fingers

Ulnar nerve

Anterior and posterior skin of little finger and half of ring finger, ulnar side of palm and back of hand

Axillary Nerve

Anterior and posterior aspects of upper arm (deltoid area)

Radial nerve

Skin of the entire posterior of arm, forearm and back of hand. Posterior skin of thumb, index, middle and 1/2 of ring fingers.

Physiology

List the 3 unique parts of a neuron	Long cell process (axon), short cell processes (dendrites), and specialized cell junctions (synapses)
What are the parts of the Synapsis?	Terminal Bouton, Presynaptic Membrane, Synaptic cleft, postsynaptic membrane, and neurosecretory vesicles
What are the types of neurons?	Bipolar (e.g. CNS cells), Unipolar (e.g. sensory neurons), and Multipolar (e.g. motor neurons)
What is myelin?	Layers of lipid-rich insulation wrapped around an axon
What is myelin's function?	To increase signal conduction speed along an axon
Which specialized support cells are responsible for myelin?	Oligodendrocytes in the Central nervous system and Schwann cells in the Peripheral nervous system
What is the space between units of myelin called?	Nodes of Ranvier
Where are nodes of Ranvier more apparent?	In the CNS. In the PNS the bare segments are partly covered by cytoplasm from Schwann cells.

True or False: One Schwann cell will produce the myelin for multiple PNS nerves' axons.	False, Oligodendrocytes in the CNS produce myelin for multiple nerves' axons, but Schwann cells in the PNS remain affixed to only one neuron's axon
What are non-neuron support cells in the CNS called?	The glia
What cells make up the glia?	Astrocytes, Oligodendrocytes, Ependyma, and Microglial cells
What are the functions of an Astrocyte?	They guide developing neurons into place during embryo development, give structure for specialized cells to exist in, and some move fluid, glucose, and ions from the local capillaries to neurons
What is the function of Ependymal cells?	They are simple cuboidal cells in the spinal cord and ventricles of the brain- that along with capillaries- form the choroid plexus. Both the choroid plexus and ependymal cells lining produce cerebrospinal fluid
What is the function of Microglia cells?	They are specialized macrophage immune cells of the CNS
From the skull moving into the brain, what are the 3 parts of the meninges?	Dura, Arachnoid, and Pia
Where do you find the main veins and arteries of the brain and the cerebrospinal fluid?	They are found in the subarachnoid space between the Arachnoid and Pia
Efferent nerves are made up of what?	Motor Autonomics
Afferent nerves are made up of what?	Sensory and Somatic
What ion is high outside the cell?	Sodium
What ion is high inside the cell?	Potassium
What establishes the electrical gradient?	Na^+/K^+ ATPase pump
How many ions are pumped in and out?	3 Na^+ out, 2 K^+ in

What is the role of the large anions trapped inside the cell?	They help generate resting membrane potential by being negative on inside compared to outside. They attract K^+ to line up on membrane on outside
What factors are necessary for establishing the resting membrane potential?	Selectively permeable membrane A gradient maintained by Na^+/K^+ ATPase pump Large anions inside cell
Influx of Na^+ into the cell such that inside becomes less negative is known as what?	Depolarization
What 2 neurotransmitters lead to depolarization?	Acytlcholine and glutamate
What two ionic events establish the phase of repolarization?	a. Na^+ stops coming into the cell (active closure of Na^+ gated channels) b. K^+ starts to slowly move out
What is Hodgkins cycle?	With a little depolarization Na^+ gated channels are open and we get an influx of Na^+ which causes more gated channels to open etc.
What stops the Hodgkins cycle?	Active closure of gated channels
What ionic event accounts for hyper-polarization, the situation in which the membrane becomes temporarily more negative than a resting membrane?	The slow closing of K^+ gated channels
The point at which an action potential is generated is known as what?	Threshold
Passive diffusion of ions through the axon providing local circuit currents is known as what?	Electrotonic conduction

What 3 factors affect membrane excitability?	a. High extracellular calcium which ↓ Na^+ influx b. A decrease in extracellular K^+ which means more K^+ will leak out down gradient via K^+ leak channels making the inside of the cell more negative and hyperpolarized c. Local anesthetics
The process in myelinated axons where the electrical conduction flows from node to node rather than down the membrane is known as what?	Saltatory conduction
What is released when an action potential reaches the terminal bouton?	Calcium
The binding of Ach to the cholinergic receptor on the post synaptic membrane causes what?	The post synaptic membrane to become permeable to Na^+ which influxes through open channels
What does acetylcholine esterase do?	It breaks down Ach thus stopping the synaptic signal
What kind of neurotransmitter causes hyperpolarization of the post synaptic membrane?	Inhibitory neurotransmitters
What 2 neurotransmitters lead to hyperpolarization?	Gama-aminobutyric acid (i.e. GABA) and glycine
Give an example of an inhibitory neurotransmitter?	GABA
What are the two precursors for Ach?	Acetyl-CoA and Choline
What breaks down norepinephrine?	Monoamine oxidase (MAO)
What ionic movement marks an inhibitory post synaptic potential? What is the net result?	Chloride into the cell Potassium out of the cell Net result is hyperpolarization
What post synaptic potential is always excitatory, always suprathreshold and always leads to an action potential?	End Plate Potential

What do we call a situation in which synapses fire at the same time in order to reach threshold?	Temporal summation
A situation in which the synapses have to be close to the axon hillock before depolarization can take place is known as what?	Spatial summation
What 3 kinds of information is supplied by sensory receptors	Type of stimuli Location of stimuli Intensity/duration of stimuli
What type of sensory receptor senses touch, pressure, position sense?	Mechanoreceptors
What type of receptors sense light?	Photoreceptors
What type of receptor senses pain?	Nociceptors
What type of receptors sense taste, smell?	Chemoreceptors
What does it mean when we say that the receptor potential is graded?	The greater the intensity of the stimulus the greater the depolarization of the sensory receptor nerve endings
The greater the amplitude of the receptor potential then the greater the frequency of action potentials up afferent nerves is known as what?	Frequency code
True or false: Receptor potentials are graded. Action potentials operate on an all or none principal.	True

Biochemistry

What nutritional deficiencies are associated with dementia and encephalopathy?	Vitamin B12, niacin, thiamine and folate
What nutritional deficiency is associated with seizures?	Pyridoxine
What nutritional deficiencies are associated with myelopathy?	Vitamin B12, Vitamin E, and folate

What nutritional deficiencies are associated with peripheral neuropathy?	Thiamine, Vitamin B12 & E, pyridoxine, and folate
What nutritional deficiencies are associated with optic neuropathy?	Vitamin B12, thiamine, and folate
What 2 biochemical reactions depend on Vitamin B12?	1. Conversion of methylmalonic acid to succinyl Co-A 2. A co-factor in the conversion of homocysteine to methionine
What is methionine used for in the nervous system?	It is converted intto S-adenosylmethioinine SAM
What other vitamin is essential in the production of methionine, SAM, and tetrahydrofolate?	Folate
Thiamine is the precursor for what co-enzyme?	Thiamine pyrophosphate, which helps produce coenzyme A
Besides Beriberi what other syndrome is associated with thiamine deficiency?	Wernicke-korsakoff syndrome
Overdose of Vitamin A results in what neurological symptoms?	Pseudotumor cerebri with headaches and papilledema
When deficient what mineral can cause myelopathy?	Copper

Pathology

What is the most common cause of infant meningitis?	*Escherichia coli*
Infection with *Clostridium botulinum* is associated with what kind of paralysis?	Flaccid paralysis
What microbe causes Lyme disease?	*Borrelia burgdorferi* (in the Americas) and *Borrelia afzeli* and *Borrelia garinii* (in Asia and Europe)
A patient comes in with fever, nausea and vomiting, stiff neck and petechiae. What is a likely diagnosis?	*Neisseria meningitidis* infection

Clostridium tetani causes what kind of paralysis?	Spastic paralysis
In what tissue can HSV-1 become latent?	The sensory ganglion cells of the dorsal root (trigeminal) ganglion, in sensory neurones
How does polio cause paralysis?	By destroying motor neurons in anterior horn and medulla
Which polio vaccine is alive attenuated and given orally?	Sabin
Which polio vaccine is inactivated multivalent and injectable?	Salk
What are the two types of leprosy?	Lepromatous and tuberculoid leprosy
Which type of leprosy is less infectious and has less bacteria?	Tuberculoid leprosy
Which type of leprosy is more infectious and has lots of bacteria present?	Lepromatous leprosy
Which type of leprosy is associated with defective cellular immunity?	Lepromatous leprosy
What happens when a neuron in the central nervous system (CNS) is damaged?	The neuron and target cell and cells targeting that neuron atrophy and die. It is not replaced and damage is permanent
What happens when a neuron in the peripheral nervous system is damaged?	The neuron will try to repair itself and restore function through a process called the axon reaction, which involves: 1. Sealing the severed ends to prevent loss of axoplasm 2. Phagocytosis of the axon and synapse distal to the damaged area by the Schwann cells 3. Filling in of the synaptic spaces by the Schwann cells 4. Sending out sprouts from the axon proximal to the cut ends which enter connective tissue and form a synapse with the target cell

What are two examples of intraneuronal bodies?	a. Pick bodies, which are dense spherical masses seen in Pick's disease b. Lewy bodies, which are densely packed fine filaments found in the brains of patients with Parkinson's disease
Neurofibrillary tangles are a type of intraneuronal body seen in the brains of what types of patients?	Patients with Alzheimer's disease, supranuclear palsy, and post-encephalitic Parkinsonism
What are the effects of glial cell reactions on the body?	a. They protect neurons and facilitate rebuilding b. They are destructive and cytotoxic when out of physiological control
What causes increased intracranial pressure?	a. Space-occupying lesions, tumors b. Hemorrhage c. Tumors d. Cerebral edema e. Hydrocephalus
What are the types of cerebral edema?	a. Vasogenic edema— caused by increased vascular permeability b. Cytotoxic edema— increase in intracellular water after cell injury, such as ischemia c. Interstitial edema— fluid accumulation in white matter with hydrocephalus
What causes hydrocephalus?	Decreased absorption or overproduction of CSF
What is the major constituent of the white matter in the CNS?	Myelin
What are the two categories into which diseases of myelin may be grouped?	a. Acquired diseases of myelin— previously normal myelin degenerates b. Hereditary myelin diseases, leukodystrophies— abnormal myelin from hereditary metabolic defects

Where are inclusion bodies found that are diagnostic features of viral infection in the brain?	a. Herpes simplex, herpes zoster, and papovavirus— found in the nucleus b. Rabies— found in the cytoplasm c. Cytomegalovirus— found in nucleus and cytoplasm
What organisms cause bacterial meningitis?	*Escherichia coli*, main cause in newborns *Haemophilus influenzae* B *Streptococcus pneumoniae*, main cause in adults *Neisseria meningitidis*, epidemic meningitis
What are the symptoms of encephalitis, a condition in which bacteria infect the brain?	Fever Nausea and vomiting with neck pain Focal neurological abnormalities Seizures Cognitive changes
What are Argyll-Robertson pupils?	A small, irregular pupil occurring in neurosyphilis in which the pupil accommodates normally with convergence but does not react to light.
What occurs with a brain abscess?	Acute inflammatory reaction and edema, followed by liquefaction necrosis, and increased intracranial pressure.
What are the subtypes of viral encephalitis?	Eastern equine Western equine St. Louis encephalitis
What is the vector for all subtypes of viral encephalitis?	Mosquitoes and birds
What viruses are known to cause viral meningitis?	Varicella zoster, Herpes simplex, HIV, influenza, and mumps

What symptoms are associated with rabies?

a. Depression
b. Malaise
c. Fever
d. Restlessness followed by uncontrollable excitement
e. Excessive salivation
f. Painful spasms of laryngeal and pharyngeal muscles
g. Exhaustion, asphyxia, general paralysis and death if not treated within 3–10 days of onset of symptoms

What structures are affected by poliovirus infection?

Motor neurons of the anterior horn of the spinal cord, medulla, cerebellum, and motor cortex.

What is a potential neurological sequelae of natural measles infection?

Subacute sclerosing panencephalitis (SSPE)

What neurological infection occurs in immunocompromised and late-stage AIDS patients?

Progressive multifocal leukoencephalopathy (PML)

What are the symptoms of Creutzfeldt-Jakob disease?

Severe, rapidly developing dementia, myoclonus, and death.

What is the most common site of cerebral infarction?

Middle cerebral artery, causing contralateral paralysis, motor and sensory defects, and aphasia.

What is the most frequent cause of intracranial hemorrhage?

Hypertension

What is a hemorrhagic stroke?

Acute bleeding into the brain tissue

What is the most common cause of subdural hematoma?

Head trauma, frequently affecting the elderly, hemophiliacs, and alcoholics.

What is an epidural hematoma?

Hemorrhage from skull fracture or blunt trauma that causes bleeding between the skull and dissected dura.

What are the symptoms of hypertension encephalopathy?

Headache and vomiting that develop into lethargy, coma and death.

What is an acute subdural hematoma?	Bleeding from bridging veins accumulating between the dura mater and arachnoid
What is the definition of a concussion?	Transient posttraumatic loss of awareness or memory that lasts seconds to minutes without causing major damage to the brain.
What are the symptoms of postconcussion syndrome?	Dizziness, depression, apathy, variable amnesia, and headaches.
What types of damage occurs to the spinal cord as a result of trauma?	a. Hemorrhage confined to cervical gray matter— lower motor neuron damage b. Laceration or transaction— loss of sensation and reflexes below level of injury, flaccid paralysis becoming spastic paraplegia c. Incomplete laceration— loss of function that depends on tract affected d. Spinothalamic tract damage— loss of temperature, pain, light or deep touch e. Posterior column damage— loss of vibration, posture, light touch
Where do tumors of the brain and brainstem occur in adults and children?	a. Adults— above the tentorium cerebelli b. Children— below the tentorium cerebelli
What are the clinical effects of neoplasms?	a. Destruction of functional neural tissue causes motor, sensory, cognitive or combination neurological deficits. b. Irritation of an area causes involuntary loss of activity, such as a seizure. c. As the neoplasm grows, its mass increases intracranial pressure and causes headaches and vomiting.
Medulloblastomas occur most frequently in what patient population?	Children

NEUROLOGICAL

What are three types of tumors of peripheral nerves?	a. Schwannomas— arising from Schwann cells b. Neurofibromatosis— arising from Schwann cells c. Von Recklinghausen's neurofibromatosis— commonly associated with café-au-lait spots
What are the symptoms of multiple sclerosis?	A variable clinical course with exacerbations and remissions, weakness of the lower extremities, visual and sensory disturbances, loss of bladder control, and mental deterioration.
What is perivenous encephalomyelitis?	An acute demyelinating disorder occurring 7–14 days after an infection or vaccination.
What often precedes Guillain-Barré syndrome?	Viral infection, immunization, or allergic reaction
What are the symptoms and characteristics of Alzheimer's disease?	a. Loss of short-term memory, progressing to loss of long-term memory b. Neuritic plaques c. Neurofibrillary tangles d. Granulovacuolar degeneration e. Atrophy of the cerebral cortex
What is the most common type of spinocerebellar degeneration?	Friedreich's ataxia, usually seen in people of European descent.
What structures are affected in Huntington's chorea?	Degeneration and atrophy of the basal ganglia and frontal cortex
What are the symptoms of Parkinson's disease?	a. Resting, pill-rolling tremor b. Masked, expressionless face c. Slow movements d. Muscular rigidity e. Shuffling gait
What occurs in amyotrophic lateral sclerosis (ALS, Lou Gehrig's disease)?	Degeneration of upper and lower motor neurons, with atrophy of skeletal muscle

What is Wernicke-Korsakoff's syndrome?	A disease, also known as alcoholic encephalopathy, that results in confusion, ataxia, and paralysis from thiamine deficiency.
What is the most common cause of vitamin B12 deficiency?	Malabsorption, particularly malabsorption caused by pernicious anemia.
What is Wilson's disease?	An autosomal recessive disease of copper metabolism causing a decrease in serum ceruloplasmin and an increase in copper in the liver, kidney, brain, and cornea.
What do storage diseases have in common?	They are all caused by autosomal recessive inborn errors of metabolism
Tay-Sachs disease most commonly affects what group of people?	Jewish families of Eastern European origin
What are the symptoms of Hurler's disease?	a. Progressive mental retardation, deterioration b. Dwarfism c. Stubby fingers d. Corneal clouding e. Early death
What are some of the causes of peripheral neuropathy?	a. Diabetes mellitus b. Uremia c. AIDS d. Nutritional deficiencies e. Mechanical compression or entrapment f. Direct trauma g. Fracture, dislocations, and penetrating injuries
What is a common example of entrapment neuropathy?	Carpal tunnel syndrome
What are the genetic characteristics of Trisomy 21 (Down's syndrome)?	Trisomy 21 is an autosomal disorder in which an additional chromosome 21 is present from abnormal egg cell meiosis

Phenylketonuria is a genetic inability (because of the lack of phenylalanine hydroxylase) to convert phenylalanine into what amino acid?

Tyrosine

Pulmonary System

Embryology

What germ layer forms the epithelial lining of the respiratory tract?	Endoderm
What is the sulcus larngotrachealis?	A groove in the ventral lower pharynx that will develop into the lungs
What is the next step in lung development?	The true lung promordium buds from the lower portion
After the true lung promordium forms, what happens next?	It divides into 2 main bronchi and the endodermal branches into the lobes
What cell is the precursor of ciliated epithelium and secretory cells in the pulmonary system?	Cubic epithelium

Anatomy

What sinus drains into the nasal cavity?	Maxillary sinus
Which meatus contains openings of maxillary and ethmoidal sinuses?	Middle meatus
What makes up the lateral walls of the nose?	The conchae
Which conch is a separate bone and contains erectile tissue?	Inferior concha

What are the 4 sinuses?	Sphenoid Frontal Maxillary Ethmoid
What arteries supply the nose?	Ant. & post. ethmoidal from the opthalmic artery Sphenopalatine and greater palatine from the maxillary artery
What is the hayfever ganglion?	Pterygopalatine ganglion mandibular division of CN V
Describe the location of the larynx by bony landmarks	Between the levels of C3-C6 vertebrae
The thyroid cartilage attaches to which cartilage?	Cricoid
What is the working cartilage of the larynx?	Arytenoid
What cartilage sits atop the arytenoid cartilage?	Corniculate cartilage
What is the space between the vocal cords called?	Rima glottidis or glottis
What is the overall source of the nerves to the larynx?	CN X (Vagus nerve)
What is in the posterior mediastinum?	Esophagus Descending aorta Azygos veins Thoracic duct Sympathetic trunk
What is in the superior mediastinum?	Aortic arch Brachiocephalic veins Phrenic nerve Vagus nerve
Foreign objects are more likely to get caught in which lung?	The right lung, because the right pulmonary bronchi is wider, shorter and more vertical than the left

What are the subdivision of the bronchial tree?	Trachea →principle bronchus →lobar bronchus →segmental bronchus →terminal bronchiole →respiratory bronchiole →alveolar duct →alveolar sac →alveolus
What adheres lung to thoracic cage, diaphragm and pericardium?	Parietal pleura
What is the thin layer over the lung called?	Visceral pleura
What is it called when you get a loss of vacuum between the visceral and parietal pleura?	Pneumothorax
What carries blood from aorta to lung tissue?	Bronchial artery
What carries blood from lung tissue to azygos veins?	Bronchial vein
What carries deoxygenated blood from right ventricle to alveoli?	Pulmonary artery
What carries oxygenated blood from alveoli to Left atrium?	Pulmonary vein
What is the location of passage of bronchi, blood vessels and nerves?	The hilum of the lung
Which lung has a horizontal fissure?	Right
The cardiac notch is found in which lung?	Left
What is the projection of the upper lobe of the left lung called?	Lingula
What nerve innervates the lungs?	CN X (Vagus nerve)
True or false: The pulmonary plexus is filled with autonomic nerve fibers that innervate the lungs?	True, the pulmonary plexus is composed of sympathetic and parasympathetic fibers that control the lungs.
What constricts bronchioles?	Parasympathetics
What dilates bronchioles?	Sympathetics
What is in the anterior mediastinum?	Thymus gland

What is in the middle mediastinum?	Heart, pericardium

Physiology

Quiet inspiration uses what to inhale?	The diaphragm
Active inspiration uses what to inhale?	Scalenes, external intercostals and SCM
Active expiration uses what to exhale?	Rectus abdominis and internal intercostals
The elastic ability of the lungs to recoil on expiration is based on what 2 factors?	Elastin Surface tension
What describes a tissues ability to distend i.e. the ability of the lungs to expand?	Compliance
What describes a tissues ability to recoil?	Elasticity
What do we have to overcome in order to inhale?	Surface tension
What substance allows the body to overcome surface tension?	Surfactant
When is the lung most likely to collapse?	End expiratory volumes
In describing the work of breathing, is rate work elastic or non-elastic?	Non-elastic
In describing the work of breathing, is depth work elastic or non-elastic?	Elastic
What describes the work required to overcome air friction in the respiratory passages?	Non-elastic work
The elastic work of the lungs has to overcome what 2 factors?	Elastic nature of tissue Surface tension
What happens with decreased compliance?	It is harder to inflate the lungs
Histamine, leukotrienes and prostaglandins have what affect on lung airway passages?	Bronchoconstriction
Sympathetic stimulation with release of epi stimulates beta 2 receptors on bronchiole smooth muscle to do what?	Relax causing bronchodilation

The rate at which new air reaches the respiratory areas is known as what?	Alveolar ventilation
The amount of air expired after quiet expiration is known as what?	Tidal volume
Maximum inspiration followed by the measurement of the volume of air expired during maximum expiration is known as what?	Forced vital capacity
Volume of air that fills the conducting passageways is known as what?	Anatomical dead space
Volume of air in respiratory areas for which no gas exchange takes place is known as what?	Physiological dead space
The amount of air expired after 1 second is measured as what?	Forced expiratory volume at 1 second (FEV1)
In what conditions do we get vasoconstriction?	Stress Inhaled irritants
The volume of air remaining in lungs after a forced expiration is known as what?	Residual volume
What nerve supplies the diaphragm?	Phrenic nerve
What respiratory center will spontaneously depolarize and allow for smooth breathing by sending signals to the phrenic nerve?	The dorsal respiratory group
What sends out inhibitory signals to the dorsal respiratory group, slowing down depolarization levels and helping set final respiratory rate and pattern?	The pneumotaxic centers
What sends signals to the accessory muscle groups leading to forced or active breathing?	Ventral respiratory groups
Where are the peripheral chemoreceptors located?	Aortic arch and carotids
What are peripheral chemoreceptors sensitive to?	Oxygen levels

With ↓ oxygen levels where does the peripheral chemoreceptor send its signal to ↑ rate of breathing?	The dorsal respiratory group
Where are central chemoreceptors located?	In the brain
What are central chemoreceptors sensitive to?	Carbon dioxide levels
What will ↑ CO_2 levels do?	They will cause the body to ↑ rate and depth of breathing
What is the major control factor of breathing?	CO_2 levels
What factors affect diffusion across the respiratory membrane?	Membrane thickness →↓ diffusion Partial pressure differences Surface area: ↓ leads to ↓ diffusion
A concept that allows us to understand respiratory exchange when there is an imbalance between alveolar ventilation and alveolar blood flow is known as what?	Ventilation/perfusion ratio which should be kept at 1 to match ventilation rate with blood flow
What is the physiological condition when the alveoli can't ventilate the amount of blood coming into the lungs?	Physiological shunt. This is where the ventilation to perfusion ratio in the lung is decreased.
What disorders set up a physiological shunt?	Lung disease (e.g. emphysema)
A situation in which there is extra air but not enough blood to oxygenate it is known as what?	Physiological dead space. The ventilation to perfusion ratio is increased in this state.
What disorders will contribute to physiological dead space? Say which side of the ratio it will affect.	Hyperventilation? ↑ alveolar ventilation, making it a physiological shunt. Pulmonary embolism? ↓ blood flow, making it a dead space.
What three things affect the oxygen-hemoglobin dissociation curve?	a. CO_2 binding →O_2 dissociates from Hgb b. H^+ ions →O_2 dissociates from Hgb c. Temperature →O_2 dissociates from Hgb

What are three ways CO_2 is carried in the body?	a. Dissolved in plasma (7%) b. Inside RBC, bound to Hgb (23%) c. In plasma as bicarbonate ion (HCO_3-) (70%)
How is respiration involved in acid base balance?	Via creation of bicarbonate that acts as a buffer in the blood: $CO_2 + H_2O \rightarrow H_2CO_3 \rightarrow H^+ + HCO_3$-

Biochemistry

In order to release carbon dioxide what must lung tissue do?	Release it from bicarbonate
Carbon dioxide is bound with a hydrogen ion to form what?	Carbonic acid
What enzyme converts carbonic acid into water and carbon dioxide?	Carbonic anhydrase
What is the structure of surfactant?	It is a lipoprotein
Respiratory mucus is composed of what?	95% water which is mostly bound with a gel containing mucins, digestive enzymes, IgA, lysozymes, electrolytes, and metabolic waste
What role do mucins play in respiratory mucus?	It protects and lubricates the tissue

Pathology

What bacteria causes pneumonia in immunocompromised patients?	*Klebsiella pneumoniae*
What causes whooping cough?	*Bordatella pertussis*
What organism causes tuberculosis?	*Mycobacterium tuberculosis*
What is the skin test for tuberculosis called?	Mantoux skin test = purified protein derivate (PPD) test = tuberculin test
What is the vaccine against tuberculosis called?	BCG, or Bacillus Calmette-Guérin
How is tuberculosis transmitted?	By respiratory droplet

What kind of immune response does the body have to tuberculosis?

Cell-mediated response, no antibodies are involved

What is tuberculosis infection that has spread to the blood called?

Miliary tuberculosis

What organism causes many cases of walking pneumonia?

Mycoplasma pneumoniae

What fungus can cause status asthmaticus?

Aspergillus

What viral pathogen with over 41 antigenic types commonly causes pharyngitis and conjunctivitis?

Adenovirus

What are the 3 main vectors for adenovirus?

Respiratory droplets
Fecal-oral routes
Direct fomite inoculation

What is allergic rhinitis?

Type I immune reaction mediated by IgE, typically causing nasal discharge

What is epiglottitis?

Life-threatening inflammation of the epiglottis, caused by H. influenzae

What are the symptoms of epiglottitis?

High fever
Drooling
Inspiratory stridor
Toxic appearance

What is the most common malignant tumor of the larynx?

Squamous cell carcinoma

What condition is associated with vocal abuse and heavy cigarette smoking?

Singer's nodule, a form of vocal cord polyps

What type of atelectasis is caused by a mass in the pleural cavity?

Compression atelectasis, which causes compression of alveoli

What type of atelectasis results from Cystic fibrosis or adult respiratory distress syndrome (ARDS)?

Patchy atelectasis

How are chronic obstructive pulmonary diseases characterized?

Physical or functional airflow obstruction

What are the four types of obstructive lung diseases?	a. Emphysema b. Chronic bronchitis c. Bronchiectasis d. Asthma
What is emphysema?	A disease resulting from enlarged alveolar spaces and increased residual volume of the lung
What is a term associated with patients with emphysema?	Pink puffers. They have to work to get air out of the lungs which results in a pink skin complexion not cyanosis.
What is the clinical definition of chronic bronchitis?	A productive cough occurring for at least three consecutive months over the course of two consecutive years
What is a term associated with patients with chronic bronchitis?	Blue bloaters. They are cyanotic due to blocked airways and systemic edema.
What is bronchiectasis?	Permanent, abnormal bronchial dilation caused by chronic infection and resulting in abundant, purulent sputum and bronchial obstruction
What is extrinsic asthma?	Childhood asthma that develops as a hypersensitivity reaction to allergens involving IgE bound to mast cells
What is the problem in restrictive lung diseases?	Decreased lung volumes and decreased compliance from conditions affecting the interalveolar septa and connective tissue
What are some types of restrictive lung diseases?	a. Pneumoconiosis b. Sarcoidosis c. ARDS d. Hypersensitivity pneumonitis e. Goodpasture's syndrome
What is adult respiratory distress syndrome (ARDS)?	Respiratory failure from simultaneous pulmonary insults, including bacterial or viral pneumonia, sepsis, chest trauma, or fat embolism.

PULMONARY

Goodpasture's syndrome is what type of hypersensitivity reaction?	Type II hypersensitivity reaction
What are the signs and symptoms of pulmonary thromboembolism?	a. Dyspnea with tachypnea b. Pulmonary hypertension with right ventricular failure c. Hyperventilation d. Arterial hypoxemia e. Pulmonary infarction
What is the number one cause of immediate death?	Death from pneumonia
What would you expect to find with bacterial pneumonia?	Consolidation, chills and fever, productive cough, blood-tinged or rusty sputum, hypoxia, shortness of breath, pleuritic pain.
What two other terms are used for primary atypical pneumonia?	Walking pneumonia Interstitial pneumonia
Ten to fifteen percent of lung abscesses are associated with what condition?	Bronchogenic cancer
What are common causes of viral pneumonia?	Adenoviruses Influenza Rubeola Varicella Respiratory syncytial virus (RSV)
What does viral pneumonia cause?	Patchy, unilateral or bilateral lobar involvement without consolidation, pleuritis or pleural effusion.
Where is histoplasmosis typically found?	Mississippi and Ohio River valleys, where it is spread by wind, birds and bats.
What does histoplasmosis mimic?	Tuberculosis
What is another name for coccidioidomycosis?	San Joaquin Valley Fever
Where is coccidioidomycosis typically found?	Southern California, southwestern U.S., northern Mexico, and parts of South America where it is spread by wind, birds and bats.

Patients with HIV infection may develop which type of pneumonia?	Pneumocystis cariniipneumonia (PCP)
What is the initial infection in tuberculosis (TB) called?	Primary tuberculosis
What is found in primary tuberculosis?	A Ghon focus, which is a single granuloma with caseous necrosis in the center and located near the pleura of one lung.
How is primary tuberculosis detected?	A positive reaction to a TB test
What occurs in secondary tuberculosis?	Ten percent of patients with primary TB develop granulomas that erode into the bronchi and bronchioles. TB may then be spread to others through aerosolized bronchial secretions.
What is the most common cause of death from cancer worldwide and in the U.S.?	Malignant carcinoma of the lung
What causes eighty-five percent of all lung cancers?	Cigarette smoking
What types of malignant neoplasms affect the lung?	Squamous cell carcinoma Large and small cell carcinomas Adenocarcinoma Bronchial carcinoid
What types of lung tumors respond to chemotherapy?	Only small cell carcinomas
What complications may occur with pneumothorax?	Negative loss of pressure of the lung may cause the mediastinum to shift and compress the other lung, creating a life-threatening situation.

Reproductive System

Embryology

What days on the menstrual cycle form the menstrual phase?	Days 1 to 4
The secretory or luteal phase occurs on what days of the menstrual cycle?	Days 15 to 28
The proliferative or follicular phase occurs on what days of the menstrual cycle?	Days 4 to 14
What hormone is released to promote the development of the follicle?	FSH
What causes a surge in LH?	Estrogen
What is the zygote?	Diploid cells resulting from union of sperm and ovum
What structure consists of 12 to 15 blastomeres?	Morula
What contains a fluid-filled cavity that separates the blastomere into two parts?	Blastula
How soon after fertilization does implantation in the endometrial epithelium of the uterus take place?	6 days
What forms the wall of the gestational or chorionic sac?	Chorion membranes
What forms the floor of the amniotic cavity?	Epiblast

What forms the roof of the exocoelomic cavity?	Hypoblast
What is the process of bilaminar embryonic disc development into trilaminar embryonic disc called?	Gastrulation
What are the three trilaminar layers called?	Ectoderm Mesoderm Endoderm
What germ layer forms the reproductive organs?	Mesoderm
What fetal organs are developed at 4 weeks gestation?	Heart Forebrain Upper and lower limbs Ears Lens of the eye
At what stage does the external auditory canal develop?	6 weeks
At what stage do the digits and external genitalia develop?	8 weeks
At what stage do the intestines develop?	7 weeks
At what stage does the ossification of bone begin?	7 weeks
True or False: Fibrocartilage forms the temporary fetal skeleton, which eventually is replaced by bone.	False, it is Hyaline cartilage
Describe the schema for fetal circulation.	Oxygenated blood from placenta via umbilical vein; through ductus venosus (bypasses the liver), into IVC and right atrium; through foramen ovale to left atrium and left ventricle, or into right ventricle to pulmonary trunk to ductus arteriosus (bypasses lungs); from aorta to internal iliac and umbilical arteries, to the capillaries in the chorionic villi of the placenta.

Anatomy

Female Reproductive Anatomy

What ligament holds ovaries to lateral wall?	Suspensory ligaments
What attaches ovaries to the uterus?	Ovarian ligament
What is the name for the peritoneum that drapes uterus, uterine tube and ovary?	Broad ligament
What is the part of the broad ligament that covers uterine tubes?	Mesosalpinx
What is the part of the broad ligament that covers the ovary?	Mesovarium
What are the names of the structures from the ovary to uterus?	Fimbriae→infundibulum→ampulla→isthmus
Where does fertilization most often take place?	In the ampulla
What ligament suspends the uterus and anchors in the labia majora via inguinal canal?	Round ligament
What female glands are homologous to the prostate gland?	Paraurethral glands
At what position on the clock are paraurethral glands located?	2 and 10 o'clock
At what position on the clock are Bartholin's glands located?	4 and 8 o'clock

Male Reproductive Anatomy

What are part of the tubule system of the testes?	Seminiferous tubules→rete testes→efferent ductules→epididymis
What structure passes through the inguinal canal?	Ductus deferens
How is the prostatic fluid secreted into the urethra?	Through the prostatic duct

What is embedded in the male external urethral sphincter?	Bulbourethral glands
Ductus deferens joins with duct from seminal vesicles to form what?	Ejaculatory duct
What are the three parts of the male urethra?	Prostatic, membronous and penile/spongy
What fills with blood during an erection?	Corpus cavernosus and corpus spongiosum
What artery is responsible for erection?	Helicine artery
The crus penis is a part of what erectile tissue?	The corpus cavernosum
The glans penis is part of what erectile tissue?	The corpus spongiosum

Physiology

What hormone will induce and maintain spermatogenesis?	FSH
What hormone promotes synthesis of testosterone from the leydig cells in testes?	LH
What substance will increase weight of testes?	FSH
What substance will stimulate sertoli cells?	FSH
What substance stimulates final maturation of the follicle?	LSH
What substance stimulates growth and initial maturation of ovarian follicle?	LH
What substance prepares follicle for action of LH?	FSH
What substance released from mature follicles inhibits FSH?	Estrogens
What substance released after ovulation inhibits FSH?	Progesterone
What substance stimulates ovulation?	LH

LH is responsible for the formation of what tissue?	The corpus luteum
What 2 hormones is LH responsible for producing via its stimulation of corpus luteum growth?	Estrogen Progesterone
What is the major androgen?	Testosterone
Where is testosterone produced?	Leydig cells
How does ↑ levels of testosterone affect spermatogenesis?	It will ↓ it due to inhibition of FSH
How is testosterone excreted?	In the bile and urine
What affect does testosterone have on sperm ducts and glands?	It is responsible for their maintenance and development
What hormone controls testosterone?	LH
What affect does testosterone have on libido?	Increases it
What is the composition of semen?	Sperm Fructose Prostaglandins Alkaline fluid
Where is estrogen secreted from in non-pregnant woman?	Corpus luteum Follicle
Where is estrogen secreted from in pregnant woman?	Placenta
What is the primary circulating form of estrogen?	Estradiol
How is estrogen excreted?	Excreted in the liver after conjugation in the liver
Proliferation and growth of reproductive tissues and secondary sexual characteristics is the function of what hormone?	Estrogen
What hormone will ↑ follicle growth?	Estrogen

What hormone will increase ovarian tube motility?	Estrogen
What hormone will inhibit secretory endometrium?	Progesterone
What effect does estrogen have on the endometrium?	Causes it to proliferate
What effect does estrogen have on breast tissue?	causes development of ducts
What effect does progesterone have on breast tissue?	It causes development of the glands
What hormone peaks before ovulation?	Estrogen
What hormone peaks after ovulation?	Progesterone
The developing follicle secretes what hormone?	Estrogen
The corpus luteum secretes what hormones?	Progesterone and estrogen
What hormone surges during the proliferative phase?	Estrogen
What hormone surges during the secretory phase?	Progesterone
Where does fertilization most often occur?	In the ampulla
What hormone stimulates the corpus luteum to still produce estrogen and progesterone?	Human Chorionic gonadotropin (HCG)
What hormone causes male fetus to secrete testosterone?	HCG
Why do estrogen and progesterone levels drop in menopause?	No follicles left to stimulate their production
What two hormones are left unopposed in menopause?	FSH and LH

REPRODUCTIVE

Biochemistry

What process gives spermatozoa ATP?	The creatine and phosphocreatine shuttle
What components make up seminal vesicle secretions?	Fructose, mucus, Vitamin C, flavins, phosphorylcholine, and protaglandins
What role does fructose play in sperm?	It is their primary fuel
What mineral is necessary for spermatogenesis?	Zinc
What components make up prostate gland secretions?	Citrate, enzymes (ex: fibrinolysin), and prostate-specific antigen
What set of vitamins may play a role in liver metabolism of estrogen?	B Vitamins
A magenisum deficiency could result in which symptoms in women?	Generalized myopathies and a lower pain thershold
What mineral effects prolactin release?	Zinc; it can inhibit prolactin release
What essential fuels or building materials are needed for endometrial growth?	Glutamine, glucose, essential fatty acids and amino acids

Pathology

What organism is most associated with toxic shock syndrome?	*Staphylococcus aureus*
How does gonorrhea usually present in males?	Urethritis, purulent discharge
What organism causes chancroid?	*Haemophilus ducreyi*
What organism is the commonest cause of epidymitis in men?	*Chlamydia trachomatis*
Which STD has a painful, ragged ulcer, and what organism causes it?	Chancroid, caused by *Haemophilus ducreyi*
What infection can be diagnosed with clue cells, and what organism causes it?	Bacterial vaginosis associated with *Gardnerella vaginalis*
How does gonorrhea present in females and what are the complications?	Usually asymptomatic, complications are PID/salpingitis and infertility

The hard chancre, a bull's eye lesion, is associated with what disease?	*Treponema pallidum* infection (syphilis)
When is syphilis infectious?	Primary and secondary infections
The mucocutaneous lesion of syphilis is found in which phase?	Secondary
The gummas appear in what stage of syphilis?	Tertiary
What is Hutchinson's triad and what is it caused by?	It is caused by congenital syphilis and has impaired vision, notched teeth and impared hearing.
Condylomata lata are associated with what disease?	Secondary, mucocutaneous lesion of syphilis
In what stage is syphilis most infectous?	Secondary stage
What sexually transmitted organism requires cholesterol and urea?	*Ureaplasma urealyticum*
What sexually-transmitted organism is associated with chronic conjunctivitis and blindness?	*Chlamydia trachomatis*
What organism causes lymphogranuloma venerum?	*Chlamydia trachomatis* serovars L1, L2 and L3
What are the most common locations for HSV-2 outbreaks?	Genitals, anus, perineum
Besides skin lesions, what is common with the initial outbreak of HSV-2?	Inguinal lymph node inflammation
What is the name for genital warts?	Condylomata acuminata cauliflower warts from HPV. Condylomata lata are flat and wart-like lesions due to secondary syphilis.
Human papillomavirus (HPV) causes what conditions?	Warts (genital and common), cervical dysplasia and cancer, anorectal cancer, squamous cell carcinoma.
Anal, oral, or genital warts are typically caused what serotypes of HPV?	HPV-6 and HPV-11

REPRODUCTIVE

Hpv-16, hpv-18 and hpv-31 are associated with what cancers?	Cervical Penile Anal
What routine test is used to detect early cervical dysplasia?	Pap smear
Does *Trichomonas vaginalis* form cysts?	No
What structure makes *Trichomonas vaginalis* motile?	Flagellum
Can *Trichomonas vaginalis* cause asymptomatic infections?	Yes, up to half of infections are believed to be asymptomatic.
Can *Trichomonas vaginalis* infect men?	Yes though less commonly than women.
What range of vaginal pH is most conducive to infection with *Trichomonas vaginalis*?	More basic than normal, roughly 5–6
What are the genetic characteristics of Turner's syndrome?	Turner's syndrome is a sex chromosome disorder in which there is an incomplete or partial chromosome 45, X genome (monosomy X), resulting in hypogonadism.
What conditions may cause vulvitis?	a. Dermatological conditions, such as psoriasis, eczema, allergic dermatitis b. Staph or strep infection
Nonspecific vulvitis may result from what conditions?	Blood dyscrasias, such as leukemia, lymphoma Uremia Diabetes
Dystrophic skin lesions often present with what symptom?	Leukoplakia
What is condyloma acuminata?	These are venereal warts, a benign hyperplasia caused by hpv types 6 and 11.
What is the most common malignant tumor of the vulva?	Squamous cell carcinoma, which is associated with hpv infection from types 16 or 18.

What is a potential sequelae of vulval intraepithelial neoplasia?	Invasive carcinoma
What is the most common form of vaginitis?	Candidiasis, a yeast infection causing a white discharge and vaginal itching.
What type of organism causing vaginitis is transmitted sexually?	Trichomonas vaginalis
The vast majority of malignant tumors of the vagina are of what type?	Squamous cell carcinoma, comprising 95% of all malignant tumors of the vagina.
What may form from chronic cervicitis?	Nabothian cysts
What are some specific causes of cervicitis?	Gonorrhea, syphilis, trichomoniasis, and candidiasis
What screening test has been effective in reducing the death rate from carcinoma of the cervix?	Papanicolaou cytologic screening test (PAP)
What is cervical carcinoma in situ?	Cervical dysplasia that reaches the basement membrane
Why is inflammation of the uterus not as common as cervicitis?	The endometrium and myometrium are resistant to disease.
What causes chronic endometritis?	Chronic PID Intrauterine devices Postpartum or post-abortion tissue retained Tuberculosis
What is adenomyosis?	Endometrium invades the myometrium in the uterus, a benign condition.
What is endometriosis?	Non-neoplastic endometrial tissue found outside the uterus, often causing bleeding and cramping.
What are chocolate cysts?	Endometriosis in the ovaries creating blood-filled cysts

What are the two forms of dysmenorrhea?	a. Primary form— no identifiable pathologic cause b. Secondary form— caused by other conditions, including chronic pelvic inflammatory disease, adenomyosis, endometriosis, fibroids
What are common causes of menorrhagia?	Endometriosis Fibroids Hormonal imbalances
What is the underlying problem in dysfunctional uterine bleeding (DUB)?	Excessive unopposed estrogen
What are leiomyomas?	Benign neoplasms that are estrogen sensitive, often causing excessive bleeding.
When does atypical endometrial hyperplasia most commonly occur?	Near menopause
What are risk factors for endometrial cancer?	Obesity Diabetes Hypertension History of anovulatory cycles
How does salpingitis most commonly present?	Acute abdomen
Of the two types of ovarian cysts, which are the most common?	Follicular cysts
Polycystic ovary syndrome (PCOS), also known as Stein-Leventhal syndrome, is associated with what signs and symptoms?	a. Bilateral cystic ovaries b. Amenorrhea c. Acne d. Dysfunctional uterine bleeding e. Insulin insensitivity f. Hypertension g. Virilism h. Hirsutism i. Infertility j. Obesity

How are ovarian cancers classified?

By the site of origin:
1. Surface
2. Epithelial
3. Germ cell
4. Ovarian sex cord-stromal tumors

How common is congenital inversion of the nipple?

Very rare, but important to be aware of when assessing for breast cancer.

What are the four basic types of fibrocystic changes that affect the breast?

a. Fibrosis form— extensive fibrous overgrowth, no epithelial hyperplasia or cysts
b. Cystic form— large spaces lined by epithelium, filled with serous fluid, blood or secretions
c. Sclerosing adenosis— firm lesions of proliferated small ducts or acini with increased stroma, no cysts
d. Ductal epithelial hyperplasia— extensive multi-layered epithelium in ducts, no cysts; premalignant

What are the signs and symptoms of bacterial mastitis?

Bacterial mastitis is a painful inflammation of the breast seen early in lactation that creates cracks and fissures in the nipples. It is usually one-sided.

What may be detected on palpation of a breast with mammary duct ectasia?

A thickened, ropey feeling from dilated ducts filled with solidified secretions.

Because traumatic fat necrosis of the breast heals with scarring and a palpable mass, it is important to distinguish it from what condition?

Carcinoma

How does fibroadenoma present?

A firm, rubbery, painless well circumscribed lesion that increases and decreases in size with menses and pregnancy.

What are the predisposing factors for breast cancer?	a. Long-term estrogen exposure due to age, late menopause, early menarche, or obesity b. No children or late birth of first child c. Previous history or family history of breast cancer d. Ductal epithelial hyperplasia
Where do most breast cancers develop?	In the ducts (90 percent)
What is intraductal carcinoma in situ (CIS)?	Malignant tumor of the duct epithelium that is not invasive and confined to the basement membrane.
What is lobular carcinoma in situ?	Non-invasive mass of abnormal cells in duct terminals, associated with fibrocystic changes or intraductal CIS.
How does Paget's disease of the breast present clinically?	It affects the nipple and areola and resembles eczema of the nipple.
What two malformations may occur to the urethral meatus of the penis?	a. Hypospadias— urethral meatus that opens on ventral surface of penis b. Epispadias— urethral meatus opens on the dorsal surface of the penis
What occurs with phimosis?	The foreskin of the penis cannot be retracted from the glans penis because of constriction. The constriction may be caused by inflammation or a congenitally narrow opening.
What inflammatory lesion of the penis is usually an acute emergency?	Paraphimosis, which blocks blood flow to the glans.
What is the most common malignant tumor of the penis?	Squamous cell carcinoma, which affects men 40 to 70 years of age and is rare in circumcised men.

REPRODUCTIVE

What conditions are known to affect the tunica vaginalis of the scrotum?	a. Hydrocele— serous fluid that fills and distends the tunica vaginalis b. Hematocele— blood that accumulates and distends the tunica vaginalis c. Chylocele— lymphatic fluid accumulation in the tunica vaginalis from elephantitis
Cryptorchidism, the failure of the testes to descend into the scrotum, is associated with what complications?	a. Testicular atrophy b. Sterility c. Increased risk of germ cell tumors
What is associated with testicular torsion?	Compromised blood supply and a hematocele
How do seminomas, the most common malignant tumor of germ cell origin, present?	Present in the testes as a painless mass of neoplastic germ cells mixed with lymphocytes.
What organism is the most frequent cause of acute prostatitis?	E.coli
What are the symptoms of both acute and chronic prostatitis?	a. Low back pain b. Dysuria c. Urgency (more common with acute prostatitis) d. Nocturia
What are the symptoms of benign prostatic hyperplasia (BPH), also known as nodular hyperplasia?	a. Frequency b. Nocturia c. Incomplete emptying of the bladder d. Hesitancy
What is the most common site of metastasis of prostate carcinoma?	Vertebrae, transported by blood and lymph

What are the stages of development of syphilis?	a. Primary syphilis begins as a hard, painless chancre b. If untreated, it goes dormant to re-emerge with symptoms including a skin rash and condyloma lata in secondary syphilis c. If left untreated, it goes dormant again and re- emerges as tertiary syphilis with many serious complications
What are the symptoms of gonorrhea in males?	Inflammation and purulent discharge
What is the most common cause of non-gonococcal urethritis?	Chlamydia
What are the symptoms of non-gonococcal urethritis?	Mild inflammation and clear discharge in males; cervicitis and clear discharge in females
How does trichomoniasis manifest in the male?	Asymptomatic; important to treat the partner so that re-infection does not occur
Hᴘᴠ may be associated with what types of cancers affecting males?	Penile and anal cancer

Urinary System

Embryology

The kidneys and the ureters arise from what germ layer?	Intermediate mesoderm
The kidneys develop from what entity?	The urogenital ridge
Of the 3 subsets of the urogenital ridge, which matures into the actual kidneys	The metanephros
From which part of the metanephros does the renal pelves, calyces, and collecting ducts develop?	The ureteric bud
The ureters develop from which portion of the metanephros?	The proximal part known as the ureteric ducts
From what germ line do the bladder and urethra develop?	Urogenital sinus

Anatomy

What rib bisects the kidney?	Rib 12
The kidneys are located between which spinal levels?	T11 - L3
What is the pathway for blood through the kidney?	Abdominal aorta→renal arteries→interlobar arteries→arcuate arteries→interlobular arteries→afferent arteriole→efferent arteriole→stellate veins→interlobular veins→arcuate veins→interlobar veins→renal veins→inferior vena cava

What is the flow of filtrate through the nephron?	Glomerulus→Bowman's capsule→proximal tubular→loop of Henle→distal tubule→collecting duct→renal pelvis
What is the muscle of the bladder?	Detrusor muscle
What is the trigone?	The 2 ureteric orifices The opening for the urethra
What nerve controls the voluntary external urethral sphincter?	Pudendal nerve S2,3,4
What effect does sympathetics have on the bladder?	Relax the detrusor muscle Activate the internal sphincter (i.e. close it off)
What effect does parasympathetics have on the bladder?	Contracts the detrusor muscle Inhibits/relaxes the internal sphincter
Where does the bladder get its blood supply?	Internal iliac artery

Physiology

What vasculature of the kidney controls glomerular blood flow?	Afferent arteriole
What controls blood flow through peritubular capillaries?	Efferent arteriole
What happens with vasoconstriction of efferent arterioles?	↑ volume of blood into glomerulus →↑ glomerular hydrostatic pressure →↑ in filtration
What is the major role of peritubular capillaries?	Reabsorption
What is the tissue that regulates the concentration of the urine?	Vasa recta
What blood vessels bring blood back to circulation?	Renal venules
What collects the filtrate?	Bowman's capsule

What part of the nephron is responsible for the majority of reabsorption?	The proximal tubule
Along with the vasa recta this part of nephron is important in controlling the concentration of urine?	The loop of Henle
Where in the nephron is filtrate monitored by osmoreceptors?	Late (convoluted) distal tubule
Which part of the nephron is impermeable to water?	Early/straight distal tubule
Which part of the nephron regulates body sodium and potassium?	Late/convoluted distal tubule
How does the body react to low Glomerular filtration rate?	a. By causing vasodilation of the Afferent arteriole with release of vasodilator substances that bind to the afferent arteriole. b. By causing vasoconstriction of efferent arteriole by release of renin which leads to angiotensin II that binds to and causes vasoconstriction of the efferent arteriole.
What are the effects of angiotensin II?	a. Local vasoconstrictor b. Promotes release of aldosterone
What stimulates renin production?	↓ in Renal Blood Flow ↓ in concentration of sodium
An indication of how effectively the kidneys clear or excrete individual substances in the blood is known as what?	Plasma clearance
What gives us a good estimate of GFR?	Plasma clearance of inulin
Substances moving passively from blood into nephron is known as what?	Filtration
Substances moving actively from blood into nephron in known as what?	Secretion
Substances moving from nephron into blood is known as what?	Reabsorption
How is water reabsorbed?	Via osmosis

Where is most of the water reabsorbed?	Proximal tubule
What follows when sodium is actively reabsorbed?	Chloride
Where in the nephron does aldosterone exert its effect on potassium and sodium?	Convoluted/late distal tubule
Where is the majority of Na^+, Cl^- and K^+ resorbed?	Proximal tubule
What injected substance is a good measure of Renal blood flow due to the fact that there is no resorption and 100% secretion?	PAH, para-aminohippuric acid
What are the effects of aldosterone?	↑ potassium secretion ↑ Sodium reabsorption H^+ excretion
What are the major controls of aldosterone?	Angiotensin II ↑ Extracellular concentration of K^+ ↓ Extracellular concentration of Na^+
Why does measuring creatinine clearance give us an overestimated estimate of GFR?	100% of creatinine that is filtered gets excreted, no reabsorption. But also a small amount gets secreted into the nephron. So final excretion is 110% of what was filtered.
Where does ADH have its effect? What is its effect?	It acts on the late/convoluted distal tubule and collecting tubule by making them permeable to water by inserting water channels into the membrane.
How is dilute urine made?	Blood osmolality is measured by osmoreceptors and the amounts of ADH are controlled accordingly. Low osmolarity and the less ADH released and the more water excreted.
An ↑ in osmolarity causes what to be released?	ADH
What controls blood osmolality?	The concentration of sodium
How does the body respond to ↑ blood osmolality?	↑ Blood osmolality is detected by osmoreceptors in the hypothalmus → release of ADH and stimulation of thirst

When do we get a craving for salt?	With low blood osmolality
When do we get a desire to drink?	With ↑ blood osmolality

Biochemistry

How is pH defined?	log 1/H+
A weak acid and its conjugate base is known as what?	A buffer
What are the 4 buffers of the body?	Bicarbonate, hemoglobin, phosphate and intracellular proteins
Generally what is the pH of the body?	Slightly alkaline at about 7.35–7.45
A substance that donates H+ is known as what?	An acid
A base is defined as?	An acceptor of H+
A solution that has the ability to resist pH changes despite added acid or base is known as what?	A buffer

Pathology

What is the most common cause of UTI?	*Escherichia coli*
Which urease-producing bacteria is often associated with UTI, especially after catheterization?	*Proteus*
Ureaplasma urealyticum causes what kind of infection?	Non-gonococcal urethritis
What are the characteristics of nephrotic syndrome?	a. Loss of negative charge on glomerular basement membranes causing proteinuria b. Generalized edema c. Hyperlipidemia d. Hypercholesterolemia
What is the most common cause of nephrotic syndrome in adults?	Membranous glomerulonephritis

Nephritic syndrome is also known by what other name?	Acute glomerulonephritis
How does nephritic syndrome manifest?	Inflammatory rupture of glomerular capillaries and bleeding, causing hematuria
Chronic glomerulonephritis may lead to what conditions?	Chronic renal failure End-stage renal disease
What is the next stage of progression with acute renal failure?	The patient may die; does not usually progress to chronic renal failure
What are the signs and symptoms of chronic renal failure?	a. Azotemia b. Metabolic acidosis c. Hyperkalemia d. Increased blood volume and hypertension e. Hypocalcemia f. Anemia
What causes tubulointerstitial nephritis?	Damage to collecting tubules and interstitium of the kidneys from drugs or toxins
What are the signs and symptoms of acute pyelonephritis?	a. Perinephric abscesses b. White blood cell casts in urine c. Urinary pain, frequency, urgency
What are the most common types of kidney stones?	Calcium oxalate Calcium phosphate Uric acid Magnesium ammonium phosphate Cystine
What types of stones fill the entire renal pelvis?	Staghorn calculi
Nephroblastoma is associated with what genetic defect?	Chromosomal deletions
Clear cell carcinoma is associated with what paraneoplastic endocrinopathies?	Polycythemia Hypercalcemia Hypertension Cushing's syndrome

Sample Exams

Anatomy Sample Exam

1. **Which of the following bones does not form part of the orbit?**
   a. Maxilla
   b. Ethmoid bone
   c. Zygomatic bone
   d. Nasal bone

2. **The atlantoaxial joint is classified as:**
   a. a pivot joint that allows uniaxial rotation of C1 around the dens axis of C2.
   b. a condyloid joint that allows uniaxial rotation of C1 around the dens axis of C2.
   c. an hinge joint that allows uniaxial flexion and extension of the head.
   d. a ball and socket joint that allows multi-axial flexion, extension, rotation of the head.

3. **The esophagus is lined by:**
   a. simple cuboidal epithelium.
   b. simple squamous epithelium.
   c. stratified squamous nonkeratinizing epithelium with mucus glands.
   d. columnar epithelium with mucus glands.

4. **The first intervertebral disc is located between:**
   a. Occiput and C1
   b. C1 and C2
   c. C2 and C3
   d. C3 and C4

5. **Which of the following statements about structures of the head is incorrect?**
   a. The temporalis muscle inserts on the coracoid process of the mandible.
   b. The coronoid process is found anterior to the mandibular notch and mandibular condyle.
   c. The mandibular foramen is found on the medial aspect of the mandible.
   d. The mental foramen is found on the lateral aspect of the mandible.

6. **Which of the following statements about the muscles of the eye is incorrect?**
   a. The tendon of the superior oblique muscle passes through a fibrous ring (trochlea) and inserts into the sclera of the eye.
   b. The eyeball is adducted by the medial rectus muscle.
   c. The eyeball medially rotated by the inferior rectus and superior rectus muscles.
   d. The inferior oblique muscle originates on the roof of the orbit.

7. **Which muscle of mastication opens (depresses) the jaw?**
   a. Temporalis
   b. Masseter
   c. Lateral Pterygoid
   d. Medial Pterygoid

8. **Which of the following muscles are not innervated by CN III?**
   a. Superior oblique and levator palpebrae
   b. Superior oblique and lateral rectus
   c. Inferior oblique and levator palpebrae
   d. Inferior oblique and superior rectus

9. **The lambdoid suture:**
   a. is found at midline between parietal bones in the median plane.
   b. represents the meeting of the frontal, parietal, temporal and sphenoid bones.
   c. divides the skull in the coronal plane between frontal and parietal bones.
   d. is the junction of the occipital and parietal bones.

10. **Which structure(s) pass(es) through the superior orbital fissure?**
    a. CNs III, IV, VI and the ophthalmic nerve (CN V_I)
    b. Optic nerve and sympathetic fibers
    c. Ophthalmic artery
    d. Internal carotid artery

11. **Which of the following are atypical cervical vertebrae?**
    a. C3-C6
    b. C1-C3
    c. C1, C2, C7
    d. C6, C7

12. **A fractured cribiform plate might result in:**
    a. pupil dilation
    b. tinnitus
    c. anosmia
    d. lateral deviation of the tongue

13. **A patient reports a loss of taste sensation which on physical exam you identify to be limited to the anterior two thirds of the tongue and palate. You are now suspecting a lesion of which nerve?**
    a. Facial nerve.
    b. Mandibular nerve.
    c. Vagus nerve.
    d. Hypoglossal nerve.

14. **What is the pathway of sound transmission from the tympanic membrane onwards?**
    a. Ossicles, round window, cochlear canals, oval window, hair cells (Organ of Corti), cochlear nerve, cochlear nuclei (medulla), superior olivary nucleus, inferior colliculus, auditory cortex (temporal lobe)
    b. Ossicles, oval window, cochlear canals, round window, hair cells (Organ of Corti), cochlear nerve, cochlear nuclei (medulla), superior olivary nucleus, inferior colliculus, auditory cortex (temporal lobe)
    c. Ossicles, oval window, cochlear canals, round window, cochlear nerve, cochlear nuclei (medulla), hair cells (Organ of Corti), auditory cortex (temporal lobe)
    d. Ossicles, oval window, cochlear canals, cochlear nerve, hair cells (Organ of Corti), round window, cochlear nuclei (medulla), auditory cortex (temporal lobe)

15. **The knee joint is:**
    a. an hinge joint between the distal end of the femur and proximal ends of the tibia and fibula.
    b. protected from posterior displacement of the femur on the tibia by the posterior collateral ligament.
    c. is most stable in the flexed position
    d. limited to about 10 degrees of medial rotation due to the winding of cruciate ligaments about each other.

16._____________**is a poorly vascularized connective tissue composed of mostly type I collagen fibers.**
    a. hyaline cartilage.
    b. elastic cartilage.
    c. fibrous cartilage.
    d. bone.

17. **The embryological umbilical vein becomes the_____________after birth:**
    a. medical umbilical ligament
    b. ligamentum venosum of the liver
    c. ligamentum teres (round ligament) of the liver
    d. round ligament of the ovary

18. **The long thoracic nerve:**
    a. innervates the rhomboids major and minor.
    b. is composed of fibres originating from anterior rami of C5, C6 and C7.
    c. traverses the glenohumeral joint.
    d. innervates the diaphragm.

19. **Which muscles make up the posterior axillary fold?**
    a. Pectoralis major and minor
    b. Serratus anterior and teres minor
    c. Latissimus dorsi and teres major
    d. Rhomboids major and minor

20. **Which artery in the Circle of Willis is unpaired?**
    a. Anterior cerebral artery
    b. Anterior communicating artery
    c. Posterior communicating artery
    d. Internal carotid artery

21. **Which wrist flexor does not pass through the carpal tunnel?**
    a. Flexor digitorum profundus
    b. Flexor digitorum superficialis
    c. Flexor pollicis longus
    d. Flexor carpi radialis

22. **Which muscle originates on the anterior sacrum and inserts on the greater trochanter of the femur?**
    a. Gracilis
    b. Piriformis
    c. Pectineus
    d. Gluteus minimus

23. **Which structure lies between the ovary and the uterine (Fallopian) tube?**
    a. Mesosalpinx
    b. Round ligament
    c. Isthmus of uterus
    d. Ligament of ovary

24. **Which of the following features of a typical vertebra is designed to restrict movement?**
    a. Spinous process
    b. Transverse processes
    c. Articular processes
    d. Vertebral arch

25. Following a recent accident your patient's radiography report indicates a fracture of the surgical neck of the humerus. Which nerve would you expect might be injured as a result of this fracture?

    a. Axillary nerve

    b. Median nerve

    c. Ulnar nerve

    d. Radial nerve

26. The lateral wall of the pelvis is formed by the___________muscle, which is innervated by the___________.

    a. piriformis; anterior rami of S1 and S2

    b. obturator internus; nerve to obturator internus

    c. coccygeus; branches of S4 and S5 spinal nerves

    d. iliococcygeus; nerve to levator ani, inferior rectal nerve and coccygeal plexus

27. Which artery exits the pelvis via the greater sciatic foramen and supplies the piriformis, tensor of fascia lata and gluteus medius and minimus muscles?

    a. Inferior gluteal artery

    b. Superior gluteal artery

    c. Internal iliac artery

    d. Internal pudendal artery

28. Which muscles help to produce flexion of the neck?

    a. Rectus capitis posterior major and minor.

    b. Longus capitis, rectus capitis anterior, suprahyoid and infrahyoid.

    c. Splenius capitis, longissimus capitis and trapezius.

    d. Rectus capitis lateralis, obliquus capitis superior and inferior.

29. Which of the following statements about the laryngeal region is incorrect?

    a. All of the intrinsic muscles of the larynx except the cricothyroid are supplied by the recurrent laryngeal nerve, a branch of CN X.

    b. The vocal ligaments extend from the arytenoid cartilage posteriorly to the anterior junction of the laminae of the thyroid cartilage.

    c. The thyroid gland lies just deep to the thyroid cartilage.

    d. The left recurrent laryngeal nerve passes inferior to the arch of the aorta.

EXAMS

30. **Which of the following statements about the lymphatics and vasculature of the lungs is incorrect?**
    a. lymphatic drainage from the parietal pleura is mainly to the lymph nodes of the thoracic wall.
    b. the right bronchial vein drains into the azygos vein, whose course is to the right of the spinal column.
    c. the two left bronchial arteries usually arise from the thoracic aorta.
    d. the pulmonary veins carry oxygen-poor blood from the lungs to the left atrium of the heart.

31. **Between which muscles do the brachial plexus and subclavian artery exit the upper thorax?**
    a. Diaphragm and the omohyoid
    b. Sternocleidomastoid and the anterior scalene
    c. Medial and posterior scalene
    d. Anterior and medial (aka middle) scalene

32. **Which of the following is not true about the Pericardium?**
    a. It lies within the superior mediastinum
    b. It is a fibroserous sac
    c. It restricts excessive movement and to lubricate the heart
    d. It extends from the second to the sixth costal cartilage

33. **The foramen ovale is found where in a fetus?**
    a. Between the umbilical vein and the inferior vena cava
    b. Between the pulmonary artery and aortic arch
    c. Between the Right and Left atrium
    d. Between the Right and Left Ventricle

34. **Which of the following arteries does not form part of the circle of Willis?**
    a. Basilar
    b. Communicating Artery
    c. Internal carotid
    d. Cerebral artery

35. **What attaches to the radial tuberosity?**
    a. Pronator Teres
    b. Latissimus dorsi
    c. Coracobrachialis
    d. Biceps brachii

Biochemistry Sample Exam

1. **Which of the following disaccharides contains an alpha-1,6 glycosidic linkage?**
   a. Sucrose
   b. Lactose
   c. Maltose
   d. Isomaltose

2. **Which of the following tissues does not depend on insulin for glucose uptake?**
   a. Liver
   b. Adipose
   c. Muscle
   d. Brain

3. **Reactions catalyzed by the enzymes hexokinase, glucokinase, PFK-1 and pyruvate kinase all require which mineral cofactor?**
   a. $Mn2+$
   b. $Mg2+$
   c. $Fe2+$
   d. $K+$

4. **The net number of ATP molecules derived from the aerobic glycolysis of one glucose molecule to (two molecules of) pyruvate is:**
   a. 10
   b. 9
   c. 8
   d. 6

5. **Which of the following statements is TRUE about glucose metabolism?**
   a. Hexokinase is inhibited by its product, glucose-6-phosphate.
   b. Liver glucokinase is inhibited by its product, glucose-6-phosphate.
   c. The lactate dehydrogenase reaction is irreversible.
   d. Pyruvate is reduced to lactate in the mitochondria

6. **The most important control of glycolysis, phosphofructokinase 1 (PFK-1):**
   a. catalyzes the conversion of glucose-6-phosphate to fructose-6-phosphate.
   b. is activated by phosphofructokinase 2 (PFK-2).
   c. is activated by fructose-2,6-bisphosphate and AMP.
   d. is most active in the "fed" state, when ATP levels are high.

7. **Which Kreb's cycle reaction requires iron as a cofactor?**
   a. Citrate synthase reaction
   b. Aconitase reaction
   c. alpha-Ketoglutarate dehydrogenase reaction
   d. Fumarase reaction

8. **Which of the following glycolytic reactions produces NADH?**
   a. Phosphofructokinase reaction
   b. Glyceraldehyde 3-phosphate dehydrogenase reaction
   c. 3-Phosphoglycerate kinase reaction
   d. Pyruvate kinase reaction

9. **Glucose can be generated:**
   a. from fatty acids via gluconeogenesis.
   b. from acetyl CoA via a direct reversal of the reactions of glycolysis.
   c. from glucose-6-phosphate via the glucokinase reaction..
   d. from glucose-6-phosphate via the glucose-6-phosphatase reaction.

10. **How do amino acids enter gluconeogenesis?**
    a. As oxaloacetate or pyruvate.
    b. As oxaloacetate only.
    c. When the dietary intake of amino acids is high, but not during starvation.
    d. Amino acids do not enter gluconeogenesis.

11. **The presence of high ATP levels would most likely:**
    a. inhibit the conversion of fructose-1,6-bisphosphate into fructose-6-phosphate via the fructose-1,6-bisphosphatase reaction of gluconeogenesis.
    b. promote the conversion of fructose-6-phosphate into fructose-1,6-bisphosphate via the PFK-1 reaction of glycolysis.
    c. inhibit the PFK-1 reaction, thereby slowing glycolysis.
    d. promote the PFK-1 reaction, thereby slowing glycolysis.

12. **Which of the following molecules can be used as precursors to glucose in gluconeogenesis?**
    a. Leucine.
    b. Lysine.
    c. Amino acids except for leucine and lysine.
    d. Fatty acids except for eicosapentaenoic acid.

13. **Products of the hexose monophosphate shunt are important in all of the following processes, except:**
    a. nucleic acid synthesis.
    b. steroid synthesis.
    c. hepatic Phase I detoxification.
    d. ketogenesis.

14. **Which of the following fatty acids directly supports the health of the colonic epithelium?**
    a. Short-chain fatty acids.
    b. Medium-chain fatty acids.
    c. Long-chain fatty acids.
    d. Trans-fatty acids.

15. **The role of HDL is to:**
    a. transport cholesterol esters from the liver to peripheral tissues.
    b. undergo endocytosis by all body cells and deliver cholesterol esters to them.
    c. remove unesterified cholesterol from peripheral tissues and deliver it to the liver.
    d. None of the above statements accurately describes the role of HDL.

16. **Which structure enters the lacteals in order to be transported to the thoracic duct?**
    a. Micelles
    b. Chylomicrons
    c. Chylomicron remnants
    d. VLDL

17. **The presence of_____________promotes optimal activity of_____________, the rate-limiting enzyme in fatty acid synthesis.**
    a. insulin; lipoprotein lipase
    b. biotin; acetyl-CoA carboxylase
    c. insulin; HMG-CoA reductase
    d. vitamin C; 7-alpha-hydroxylase

18. **What is the biologically active form of vitamin D?**
    a. 25-hydroxy-D_3
    b. 24, 25-dihydroxy-D_3
    c. 7-dehydrocholesterol
    d. Calcitriol

19. **Which of the following amino acids is non-essential?**
    a. Tryptophan
    b. Tyrosine
    c. Threonine
    d. Methionine

20. **Free vitamin B12:**
    a. is easily obtained in the diet.
    b. requires intrinsic factor (IF) for absorption.
    c. is most commonly found in supplements.
    d. is absorbed by the gastric parietal cells.

21. **The body's major intracellular cation is:**
    a. $Ca2+$
    b. $Mg2+$
    c. $Na+$
    d. $K+$

22. **Cholesterol is not a precursor of:**
    a. bile acids.
    b. globulin.
    c. vitamin D.
    d. adrenocorticosteroids.

23. **Uric acid is a product of the degradation of:**
    a. cytosine and thymine.
    b. thymine and uracil.
    c. adenine and uracil.
    d. adenine and guanine.

24. **The process of _____________ occurs in the _____________ under the influence of steroid hormones.**
    a. DNA replication; cytoplasm
    b. transcription; nucleus
    c. translation; nucleus
    d. post-translational modification; cytoplasm

25. **What is the rate-limiting step in essential fatty acid metabolism?**
    a. Delta-6 desaturase
    b. Elongase
    c. HMG-CoA reductase
    d. Thiolase

26. Which of the following is not a fat-soluble vitamin?

    a. Menaquinone

    b. Calcitriol

    c. Retinol

    d. Pyridoxal

27. Which of the following substances allows for biliary excretion of bilirubin?

    a. Biliverdin

    b. Glucuronic acid

    c. Glutathione

    d. Heme

28. Allosteric regulation of enzyme activity is characterized by:

    a. proenzyme activation.

    b. increased transcription of the genes that code for the enzyme.

    c. non-covalent binding to modify the shape of the enzyme.

    d. covalent modification by phosphorylation or dephosphorylation.

29. An enzyme that catalyses the transfer of a phosphate group is considered to be a:

    a. kinase.

    b. phosphatase.

    c. transaminase.

    d. protease.

30. Which of the following substances is not used by the liver in the production of urea?

    a. Ammonia

    b. Aspartate

    c. Alanine

    d. Carbon dioxide

31. Which of the following is not a Ketone body?

    a. acetone

    b. butyraldehyde

    c. acetoacetate

    d. beta-hydroxybutyrate

32. To transport ____________into the mitocondria for Beta oxidation __________is needed.

    a. Malonyl SCoA; carnitine

    b. Acyl SCoA; carnitine

    c. Acyl SCoA; taurine

    d. Malonyl SCoA; taurine

33. What co-factors are necessary for the delta-6-desaturase conversion of linoleic acid to gamma-linolenic acid?

    a. thiamin, cobalamin, Zinc, Magnesium

    b. niacin, cobalamin, Vitamin C, and biotin

    c. riboflavin, thiamin, niacin, pyridoxine

    d. niacin, pyridoxine, Vitamin C, Zinc, and Magnesium

Pathology Sample Exam

1. Cellular injury due to the immune system's response to a microbial infection is termed:

    a. immunological injury.

    b. infectious injury.

    c. reversible injury.

    d. chemical injury.

2. Which one of the following statements about apoptosis is true?

    a. Apoptosis is inducible by DNA injury and suppressible by cytokines.

    b. Apoptosis in a cluster of cells tends to induce an inflammatory response in adjacent cells.

    c. Apoptosis is most active in malignant cells.

    d. Apoptosis normally occurs in tissue cultures after about 7 cell divisions.

3. The presence of excess bilirubin in the blood is associated with:

    a. hemochromatosis and hemosiderosis.

    b. jaundice and erythrocyte destruction.

    c. the normal aging process.

    d. tyrosine oxidation and UV light exposure.

4. Chronic inflammation is typically characterized by the presence of:

    a. neutrophils, swelling and vasodilation.

    b. neutrophils, angiogenesis and fever.

    c. macrophages, angiogenesis and fibroblasts.

    d. macrophages and neutrophils.

5. Which of the following signs/symptoms characterize irreversible shock?

    a. hypoxia and alkalosis.

    b. increased respiratory rate and heart rate..

    c. peripheral vasodilation.

    d. tubular necrosis and renal failure.

6. **Sickle cell anemia is an example of which type of genetic mutation?**
   a. Point mutation.
   b. Deletion.
   c. Insertion.
   d. Trinucleotide repeat.

7. **Which of the following pathologies is characterized by antibody-producing plasma cells, lytic bone lesions and renal failure?**
   a. Chronic myelogenous leukemia.
   b. Chronic lymphocytic leukemia.
   c. Acute lymphocytic leukemia.
   d. Multiple myeloma.

8. **A vitamin K deficiency will impede the synthesis of which of the following clotting factors?**
   a. von Willebrand's factor.
   b. Factor VIII.
   c. Prothrombin and factors VII, IX, X.
   d. Fibrinogen.

9. **Hodgkin's lymphoma most commonly affects young men and is characterized by the presence of:**
   a. Bence-Jones proteins.
   b. Reed-Sternberg cells.
   c. X-linked recessive inheritance.
   d. Koplik's spots.

10. **The finding of immune complex deposits and fibrosis in arterial walls within visceral organs as well as segmental loss of arterial lumen would support the diagnosis of:**
    a. Raynaud's phenomenon
    b. Raynaud's disease
    c. thromboangitis obliterans
    d. polyarteritis nodosa

11. **Which of the following venous pathologies is the most dangerous?**
    a. Varicosities of the superficial veins of the legs.
    b. Esophageal varices.
    c. Anal hemorrhoids.
    d. Rectal hemorrhoids.

EXAMS

12. **Which one of the following cardiac features is not found in the Tetralogy of Fallot?**
    a. Pulmonary stenosis.
    b. Left ventricular hypertrophy.
    c. Overriding aorta.
    d. Ventricular septal defect.

13. **A concerned parent brings her 26-month old male child into your office after an apparent worsening of his cold symptoms. The child appears "toxic" and has a temperature of 39° C or 102.2° F. You notice an inspiratory stridor and that the child is drooling. Which of the following pathologies do you most strongly suspect?**
    a. Laryngitis.
    b. Laryngeal cancer.
    c. Epiglottitis.
    d. Vocal cord polyps.

14. **In the above case, what is the most likely etiology of the child's illness?**
    a. Inflammation of the epiglottis caused by H. influenzae infection.
    b. Irritation of the vocal cords due to excessive crying.
    c. Exposure to second-hand smoke in the home.
    d. Inflammation of the larynx due to viral infection.

15. **K.S, a 38-year-old male bank teller, presents to your clinic with a chief complaint of difficulty breathing and joint pain. On physical exam, you notice lymphadenopathy of his cervical and inguinal lymph nodes. K.S. has an oral temperature of 37.9° C or 100° F and shows a slightly blue complexion. His respiration rate is 24 breaths per minute, with no wheezing or stridor. His history is negative for allergies, smoking and occupational dust exposure. Which of the following respiratory pathologies would you most strongly suspect in this patient?**
    a. Restrictive lung disease; pneumoconiosis
    b. Restrictive lung disease; sarcoidosis
    c. Obstructive lung disease; asthma
    d. Obstructive lung disease; emphysema

16. **Visualizing small white spots on a red base on the surface of your patient's oral mucosa, which of the following etiologies is most indicated?**
    a. Measles infection
    b. Herpes simplex infection
    c. Poor oral hygiene
    d. Chronic use of chewing tobacco

17. **Pancreatic cancer localized at the head of the pancreas may obstruct the common bile duct, resulting in:**
    a. impaired bilirubin conjugation.
    b. impaired bilirubin synthesis.
    c. hemolytic jaundice.
    d. obstructive jaundice.

18. **Thickening of the glomerular basement membrane can lead to urinary protein loss and generalized edema, as in:**
    a. nephrotic syndrome.
    b. nephritic syndrome.
    c. nephrosclerosis.
    d. acute pyelonephritis.

19. **Which type of renal stone would be most likely to form in the presence of urea-splitting bacteria, which permanently alkalinize the urine?**
    a. Calcium oxalate
    b. Calcium phosphate
    c. Struvite (calcium, magnesium and ammonium phosphates)
    d. Cystine

20. **Which of the following clinical scenarios can lead to hydronephrosis?**
    a. Obstruction of the renal pelvis by calculi or tumors.
    b. Compression of the ureters during pregnancy.
    c. Compression of the urethra due to prostatic hyperplasia or carcinoma.
    d. All of the above scenarios can lead to hydronephrosis.

21. **The most common malignant tumor of the vulva, ____________is often associated with infection with HPV types ____________.**
    a. carcinoma in situ; 6 and 11
    b. condylomata acuminata; 6 and 11
    c. condylomata lata; 16 and 18
    d. squamous cell carcinoma; 16 and 18

22. **What is the most common tumor of the female reproductive system?**
    a. Leiomyoma.
    b. Leiomyosarcoma.
    c. Squamous cell carcinoma.
    d. Condyloma.

23. Inflammation of a retracted, phimotic foreskin is termed ______________, and should be managed.

   a. epispadias; surgically.

   b. phimosis; with improved hygiene practices.

   c. paraphimosis; as an acute emergency.

   d. balanoposthitis; with antibiotics.

24. What is the most common cause of male urinary tract obstruction?

   a. Benign prostatic hyperplasia.

   b. Cryptorchidism.

   c. Sertoli cell tumor.

   d. Calcium oxalate stones.

25. Which microorganism is the most common cause of non-gonococcal urethritis?

   a. Chlamydia trachomatis

   b. Trichomonas vaginalis

   c. Neisseria gonorrhea

   d. Treponema pallidum

26. Hypoadrenalism caused by suppression of ACTH secretion by exogenous administration of steroids is termed:

   a. Addison's disease.

   b. Cushing's syndrome.

   c. Waterhouse-Friderichsen syndrome.

   d. Secondary adrenocortical insufficiency.

27. Rheumatoid arthritis is most commonly characterized by:

   a. past medical history of Lyme disease orNeisseria gonorrhea infection.

   b. progressive rigidity of the lumbar spine and the presence of HLA-B27.

   c. chronic bilateral inflammation of PIP and MCP joints, ulnar wrist deviation and the presence of HLA-DR4.

   d. bone spurs, Heberden's nodes on DIP joints and Bouchard's nodes on PIP joints.

28. Which of the following skeletal pathologies is least likely to affect an elderly patient?

   a. Osteoporosis.

   b. Osteitis deformans.

   c. Osteosarcoma.

   d. Osteomalacia.

29. Which of the following autoimmune diseases is characterized by autoantibody-mediated destruction of the salivary and lacrimal glands?

    a. Systemic lupus erythematosis.

    b. Sjøgren's syndrome.

    c. Scleroderma.

    d. Sclerodactyly.

30. Which pathological finding is typical of Alzheimer's disease?

    a. Lewy bodies.

    b. Neurofibrillary tangles.

    c. Negri bodies.

    d. Homer-Wright rosettes.

31. Hirshsprung's disease is due to a failure to develop what?

    a. Auerbach's plexus

    b. Meissner's plexus

    c. Tegmental fibers

    d. Both a and c

32. Which of these would be signs of a Hypoglossal nerve lesion?

    a. Paralysis of the Sternocleidomastoid muscle

    b. Tongue deviates towards affected side

    c. Tongue muscle atrophy to unaffected side

    d. A loss of ability to taste sweet, salty, sour or bitter on the anterior 2/3 of the tongue

33. In Parkinson's disease which parts of the brain degenerate?

    a. Substantia nigra

    b. Basal nuclei

    c. Pallidorungal fibers

    d. Amygdala

34. Which of these is not responsible for limiting or controlling acute inflammation?

    a. Fibrinolysis

    b. Kinin system

    c. Coagulation

    d. Complement system

35. A 63yoa male presents with episodes of intense sharp and stabbing pains on his left side near his cheek, eye, and chin. Each episode only lasts a few seconds and is triggered by brushing his teeth, chewing, or touching his face on the left. All finding are normal on a neurological, optic, and auditory examination. The most likely diagnosis is what?

    a. Temporomandibular joint dysfunction

    b. Temporal arteritis

    c. Post-herpetic neuralgia

    d. Trigeminal neuralgia

Physiology Sample Exam

1. Vitamin D is required for the active absorption of which mineral?

    a. Sodium

    b. Potassium

    c. Iron

    d. Calcium

Marieb (2004). P. 931

2. What is the major regulator of PTH secretion?

    a. Plasma [Ca2+]

    b. Plasma [phosphate]

    c. Vitamin D

    d. The kidneys

Boron & Boulpaep (2005). Medical Physiology Updated Ed. p. 1090

3. What is the correct sequence of steps involved in muscle relaxation?

    A. Ca++ is actively pumped back into the sarcoplasmic reticulum.

    B. The muscle fiber returns to its resting length as the thick and thin myofilaments are disconnected.

    C. Tropomyosin shifts back to occupy the active sites of actin.

    D. Myosin cross bridges are prevented from binding to actin.

    a. A, C, D, B

    b. A, B, C, D

    c. C, A, B, D

    d. C, D, A, B

Thibodeau & Patton (2003). Anatomy & Physiology Fifth Ed. Mosby. p. 316

4. **What does the QT interval of an electrocardiogram represent?**
   a. Atrial depolarization
   b. Ventricular repolarization
   c. Ventricular depolarization and repolarization
   d. Conduction velocity through the AV node

   Costanzo (2007). Physiology 4th Ed. Lippincott Willians & Wilkins. p.73

5. **An ileectomy that resulted in the loss of 95% of the ileum might lead to the development of _____________.**
   a. Pernicious anemia
   b. Achlorhydria
   c. Hypochlorhydria
   d. Intrinsic factor defiency

   Costanzo (2007). Physiology 4th Ed. Lippincott Willians & Wilkins. p.227

6. **Which of the following statements about regulation of sodium balance is TRUE?**
   a. Aldosterone is released in response to sympathetic stimulation, decreased filtrate osmolality or decreased stretch at the juxtaglomerular apparatus.
   b. Renin catalyzes the production of angiotensin II.
   c. Decreased K+ levels in the ECF stimulate aldosterone release.
   d. Active reabsorption of Na+ by the distal convoluted tubules and collecting ducts is highest when aldosterone levels are low.

7. **During the menstrual phase of the uterine cycle:**
   a. ovarian hormones are at their highest levels.
   b. gonadotropin levels are beginning to rise.
   c. the endometrium becomes thick and well-vascularized.
   d. estrogens induce synthesis of progesterone receptors in endometrial cells.

   Marieb (2004). p. 1093

8. **Calcium deficiency may typically lead to any of the following physiological states EXCEPT:**
   a. muscle tetany.
   b. osteomalacia.
   c. osteporosis.
   d. kidney stones.

   Marieb (2004). P. 951

9. A patient with a history of severe renal disease presents with tremors, muscle weakness, irregular heartbeat and hypertension. You suspect this patient may have a:

   a. sodium deficiency.

   b. magnesium deficiency.

   c. chromium excess.

   d. chloride excess.

    Marieb (2004). P. 951–952

10. A patient tells you she has noticed increasing numbness and loss of sensation in her hands and feet since her last visit several months ago. You notice that she has some difficulty walking into your office, and that her deep tendon reflexes are depressed. Sensing she may have misunderstood your last prescription for B-vitamins, what condition do you immediately suspect?

   a. biotin deficiency

   b. vitamin B6 excess

   c. vitamin B12 excess

   d. folate deficiency

    Marieb (2004). P. 949–950

11. The presence of fatty chyme in the duodenal mucosa signals the secretion of . . . Marieb (2004) p. 905

   a. CCK (cholecystokinin), which triggers pancreatic secretion and gall bladder contraction.

   b. somatostatin, which inhibits pancreatic secretion and gall bladder contraction.

   c. histamine, which signals the parietal cells to release HCl.

   d. serotonin, which causes stomach muscle contraction.

12. Which of the following statements is *true* about the body's handling of iron?

   a. Iron absorption occurs at a constant rate, irrespective of the body's need for iron.

   b. Menstrual bleeding is not a significant cause of iron loss for females.

   c. Ionic iron is actively transported into intestinal mucosal cells, where it is bound to ferritin and locally stored.

   d. Iron is transported in the circulation by the plasma protein, hemosiderin.

    Marieb (2004) p. 931

13. What renal effect would be expected in a state of dehydration?

   a. Increased glomerular osmotic pressure and increased filtrate formation.

   b. Increased glomerular osmotic pressure and decreased filtrate formation.

   c. Increased glomerular hydrostatic pressure and increased GFR.

   d. Increased glomerular hydrostatic pressure and decreased GFR.

    Marieb (2004) p. 1007

14. How does kidney tubular secretion influence acid-base balance in the body?

    a. When the blood becomes too acidic, the renal tubule cells actively secrete more HCO_3^- and K+ into the filtrate and retain more Cl-.

    b. When the blood becomes too acidic, the renal tubule cells actively secrete more H+ into the filtrate and retain more HCO_3^- and K+.

    c. When the blood becomes too alkaline, the renal tubule cells actively secrete more H+ into the filtrate and retain more Cl-

    d. Tubular secretion does not significantly affect acid-base balance in the body. Ref: Marieb (2004) P. 1014.

15. A blood sample from a patient with a history of allergies would show a higher than normal proportion of:

    a. neutrophils.

    b. erythrocytes.

    c. eosinophils.

    d. natural killer cells.

Marieb (2004). Human Anatomy & Physiology. P. 656–657.

16. The defecation reflex is:

    a. not influenced by conscious control by the cerebral cortex.

    b. completely under conscious control by the cerebral cortex.

    c. a sympathetic spinal cord reflex that causes smooth muscle relaxation in the rectal walls.

    d. a parasympathetic spinal cord reflex that causes the rectum to contract and the anal sphincters to relax.

Marieb (2004). P. 925

17. The most important function of the mineralocorticoids is to:

    a. regulate extracellular electrolyte concentrations.

    b. enhance resistance to stress.

    c. promote bone mineralization.

    d. control blood glucose levels.

18. How is bilirubin transported in the blood?

    a. Bound to ligandin.

    b. Bound to albumin.

    c. As free bilirubin.

    d. As urobilinogen.

19. **Which hormone promotes milk release during lactation?**
    a. Oxytocin
    b. Prolactin
    c. Estrogen
    d. Human chorionic gonadotropin

20. **Which of the following responses is not considered to be an adaptive effect of exercise?**
    a. Decreased insulin sensitivity.
    b. Increased mitochondria.
    c. Decreased risk of injury.
    d. Increased white blood cell count.

21. **Body temperature homeostasis does not involve:**
    a. Sympathetic input to the sweat glands.
    b. Sympathetic input to the blood vessels of the skin.
    c. Involuntary motor input to the skeletal muscles.
    d. Afferent input from peripheral and central thermoreceptors to the pituitary gland.

22. **Which of the following factors would shift the hemoglobin oxygen saturation curve to the right (i.e. causing hemoglobin to unload more oxygen to the tissues)?**
    a. Decreased body temperature.
    b. Exercise.
    c. Decreased [2,3-bisphosphoglycerate].
    d. Higher pH.

23. **Cardiac muscle cells:**
    a. are multinucleated.
    b. are spindle-shaped.
    c. contain few mitochondria.
    d. are electrically coupled via gap junctions.

Marieb (2004). P. 687

24. **Which of the following muscles does not assist in forced expiration?**
    a. Internal intercostals
    b. Transverse and oblique abdominal muscles
    c. Latissumus dorsi
    d. Scalenes

Marieb (2004). P. 846–847

25. The volume of air that can be forcibly inspired beyond the tidal volume is called the:
   a. inspiratory reserve volume (IRV).
   b. residual volume (RV).
   c. functional residual capacity (FRC).
   d. total lung capacity (TLC).

26. A patient presents with new difficulty in producing speech but seems to have normal language comprehension. You suspect a lesion affecting:
   a. Wernicke's area.
   b. Broca's area.
   c. The lateral prefrontal cortex.
   d. The lateral and ventral parts of the temporal lobe.

Marieb (2004). P. 441

27. Fast glycolytic muscle fibers:
   a. are large and pale, contract rapidly and are substantially supplied with mitochondria.
   b. are red, intermediate in size and are high in myoglobin.
   c. contract powerfully and are prone to fatigue and lactic acid accumulation.
   d. contract slowly and are fatigue-resistant.

28. Vitamin K is required for the synthesis of which coagulation factor(s)?
   a. I, II, III
   b. II, VII, IX, X
   c. von Willebrand factor (vWF)
   d. Thromboxane A_2 (TXA$_2$)

29. Which statement is TRUE about gastric secretion?
   a. Parietal cells in the fundus secrete gastrin, ACh and histamine in response to HCl.
   b. Mucous cells in the antrum secrete pepsinogen and mucus in response to vagal (ACh) stimulation.
   c. Chief cells in the fundus secrete pepsinogen in response to NE.
   d. G cells in the antrum secrete gastrin in response to somatostatin.

Ref: Costanzo (2007). Physiology 4th Ed. Lippincott Willians & Wilkins. p.214

30. Which of the following physiologic states might lead to peripheral edema?
   a. Systemic hypertension.
   b. Increased capillary oncotic pressure.
   c. Excessive lymphatic drainage of fluid from the interstitium.
   d. Hyperproteinemia.

31. **A patient comes in complaining of a loss of taste. Which Cranial nerves would you suspect are involved?**
    a. CN IX and CN VII
    b. CN IX and CN V
    c. CN XII and CN V
    d. CN XII and CN VII

32. **What respiratory cell plays a part in blood pressure regulation?**
    a. Type II cells
    b. Type I cells
    c. Pseuodostratified columnar cells
    d. Goblet cells

Microbiology Sample Exam

1. **Which of the following is not one of the cardinal signs of inflammation?**
    a. Pallor
    b. Heat
    c. Pain
    d. Swelling

2. **An infection acquired due to hospitalization is considered to be:**
    a. nosocomial
    b. iatrogenic
    c. zoonotic
    d. latent

3. **Which one of the following microorganisms typically causes bloody diarrhea?**
    a. Clostridium perfringens
    b. Yersinia enterocolitica
    c. Enterotoxigenic *E. coli* (ETEC)
    d. Enteropathogenic *E. coli* (EPEC)

4. **The exotoxin of *Clostridium botulinum* acts at/on the ___________, resulting in ___________.**
    a. endothelium; cell lysis
    b. epidermis; skin rash
    c. neuromuscular junction; flaccid paralysis
    d. neurones; spastic paralysis

5. "Rose spots" is a typical feature of _____________, caused by _____________ infection.
   a. Scarlet fever; *Streptococcus pyogenes*
   b. Syphilis; *Treponema pallidum*
   c. Typhoid; *Salmonella typhi*
   d. Typhus; *Rickettsia prowazeki*

6. **With respect to *Streptococcus* spp., which of the following statements is incorrect?**
   a. *Strep. agalactiae* (Group BStrep.) normally colonizes the human respiratory tract.
   b. *Strep. pyogenes* is susceptible to penicillin.
   c. Rheumatic fever is one of the possible sequelae ofStrep. pyogenes infection.
   d. Strep. mutans causes dental caries.

7. **Which of the following herpes viruses can cause gastroenteritis?**
   a. Human herpes virus-6
   b. Herpes simplex II
   c. Adenovirus
   d. Human papillomavirus

8. **Maternal infection with which of the following viruses is not considered a risk to a developing fetus?**
   a. Parvovirus B19
   b. Rubivirus (rubella virus)
   c. Cytomegalovirus
   d. Rhinovirus

9. **Which of the hepatitis viruses can produce a carrier state?**
   a. A and B
   b. B and C
   c. A and D
   d. D and E

10. ***Cryptosporidium parvum* infection is characterized by:**
    a. malaria
    b. fetal transmission
    c. arthritis
    d. diarrhea

For questions 11 and 12, consider the following case:
Your 20-year-old male patient presents to your clinic with weight loss and fatigue following his return five weeks ago from a tour of Central America. He tells you that in the last week of his trip he ate a pork stew that hadn't seemed "properly cooked". A stool sample was negative for a panel of enteropathogenic bacteria.

11. **Which of the following parasitic microorganisms do you suspect this patient may be infected with?**
   a. *Trypanosoma cruzi*
   b. *Taenia solium*
   c. Togavirus
   d. *Toxoplasma gondii*

12. **Which of the following clinical manifestations might be discovered on further evaluation of this patient?**
   a. Cysticercosis
   b. Perianal itching
   c. Gastroenteritis
   d. Elephantiasis

13. **Which of the following microorganisms is not a normal part of the microflora of human skin?**
   a. *Staph. aureus*
   b. *Staph. epidermidis*
   c. *Pseudomonas aeruginosa*
   d. *Bacillus anthracis*

14. **A 51-year-old craftsman presents to your clinic with fever, hypotension and a macular erythematous rash with some areas of desquamation. His history is unremarkable except for a recent hand wound due to an accident in his workshop. This wound has remained painful and is showing signs of infection. You ascribe his symptoms to:**
   a. erysipelas caused by *Strep. pyogenes*
   b. toxic shock syndrome caused by *Staph. aureus* exotoxins
   c. cellulitis caused by *Strep. pyogenes* infection
   d. impetigo caused by *Strep. pyogenes* and/or *Staph. aureus*

15. **Which of the following gram-negative curved rods typically cause food poisoning?**
   a. *H. pylori* and *Vibrio cholerae*
   b. *Campylobacter jejuni* and *Vibrio cholerae*
   c. *H. pylori* and *Vibrio parahemolyticus*
   d. *Campylobacter jejuni* and *Vibrio parahemolyticus*

16. **Chancroid is characterized by:**
   a. soft, painful, genital lesions due to *Haemophilus ducreyi* infection
   b. soft, painful, genital lesions due to *Haemophilus influenzae* infection
   c. hard, painless genital lesions due to *Treponema pallidum* infection
   d. soft, painful, genital lesions due to HPV infection

17. A 26-year-old, sexually active female presents with copious, foul-smelling vaginal discharge. Microscopic examination of the discharge shows motile trophozoites, confirming your diagnosis of:

  a. *Gardnerella vaginalis* infection
  b. *Trichomonas vaginalis* infection
  c. *Candida* infection
  d. *Ureaplasma urealyticum* infection

18. _____________ infection is the most common cause of infant pneumonia and is transmitted by ______________.

  a. Respiratory syncytial virus; respiratory droplets
  b. *Mycoplasma pneumoniae*; respiratory droplets
  c. *Chlamydia* (Chlamydophila) *trachomatis*; respiratory tract colonization during birth
  d. *Legionella pneumophila*; contaminated ventilation systems

19. A lymph node biopsy from an otherwise healthy adult resident of the central U.S. who has presented with an acute fungal pulmonary infection would most likely confirm the presence of ______________.

  a. *Candida albicans*
  b. *Pneumocystis carinii*
  c. *Histoplasma capsulatum*
  d. *Aspergillus* spp.

20. Which of the following gram-positive bacilli is not spore-forming?

  a. *Bacillus cereus*
  b. *Corynebacterium diphtheriae*
  c. *Clostridium tetani*
  d. *Clostridium perfringens*

21. Which of the following gram-negative rods does not have a flagellum for motility?

  a. *Campylobacter jejuni*
  b. *Shigella* spp.
  c. *Vibrio cholerae*
  d. *Pseudomonas aeruginosa*

22. Which human prion disease is linked with consumption of BSE (bovine spongiform-encephalopathy)-infected food?

  a. Creutzfeldt-Jacob disease
  b. Variant Creutzfeldt-Jacob disease
  c. Kuru
  d. Scrapie

23. Which of the *Staphylococcus* spp. produces coagulase and exotoxins?

    a. *Staph. aureus*

    b. *Staph. epidermidis*

    c. *Staph. saprophyticus*

    d. All *Staph.*spp. produce coagulase and exotoxins.

24. Which of the following gram-positive cocci are beta-hemolytic on blood agar and can cause meningitis and septicemia in neonates?

    a. *Strep. pneumoniae*

    b. *Strep. mutans*

    c. *Strep. agalactiae*

    d. *Enterococcus faecalis*

25. How does *H. pylori* frespond to gastric acid?

    a. *H. pylori* uses gastric acid to initiate gastric neoplasia.

    b. *H. pylori* produces a toxin that is activated by gastric acid and produces ulceration.

    c. *H. pylori* secretes protease, which produces bicarbonate to buffer gastric acid.

    d. *H. pylori* secretes urease, which produces ammonia to buffer gastric acid.

26. Lymphocytes are derived from:

    a. stem cells in the bone marrow and thymus.

    b. stem cells in the spleen.

    c. MALT (mucosa-associated lymphoid tissue).

    d. the lymph nodes.

27. Which of the following statements best describes the roles of interferons (IFN) and tumor necrosis factor (TNF-alpha):

    a. IFNs and TNF-alpha are both derived from monocytes and T cells.

    b. IFNs and TNF-alpha have antiviral activity.

    c. IFNs are antiviral and TNF-alpha is involved in cytotoxicity, cachexia and fever.

    d. TNF-alpha is antiviral and IFNs are involved in cytotoxicity, cachexia and fever.

28. Which immunoglobulin type is produced by the MALT (mucosa-associated lymphoid tissue) for mucosal secretions?

    a. IgA

    b. IgG

    c. IgE

    d. IgM

29. Immunological memory:
  a. produces a stronger, faster response to a given antigen as compared to the primary immune response.
  b. produces a weaker, slower response to a given antigen as compared to the primary immune response.
  c. engages B cells but not T cells.
  d. engages T cells but not B cells.

30. A few weeks after an acute streptococcal infection a patient's urine sample is showing albumin and red blood cells. You will need to rule out acute glomerulonephritis caused by which type of hypersensitivity reaction?
  a. Type I, allergic reaction to streptococcal antibodies
  b. Type II, glomerular cytotoxicity induced by IgG antibodies
  c. Type III, glomerular deposition of immune complexes containing streptococcal antigens
  d. Type IV, cell mediated response to streptococcal antigens in the flomerulus

31. *Campylobacter jejuni* has been associated with the development of what condition?
  a. Guillain-Barré
  b. Myasthenia gravis
  c. Lyme Disease
  d. Poryphyric neuropathy

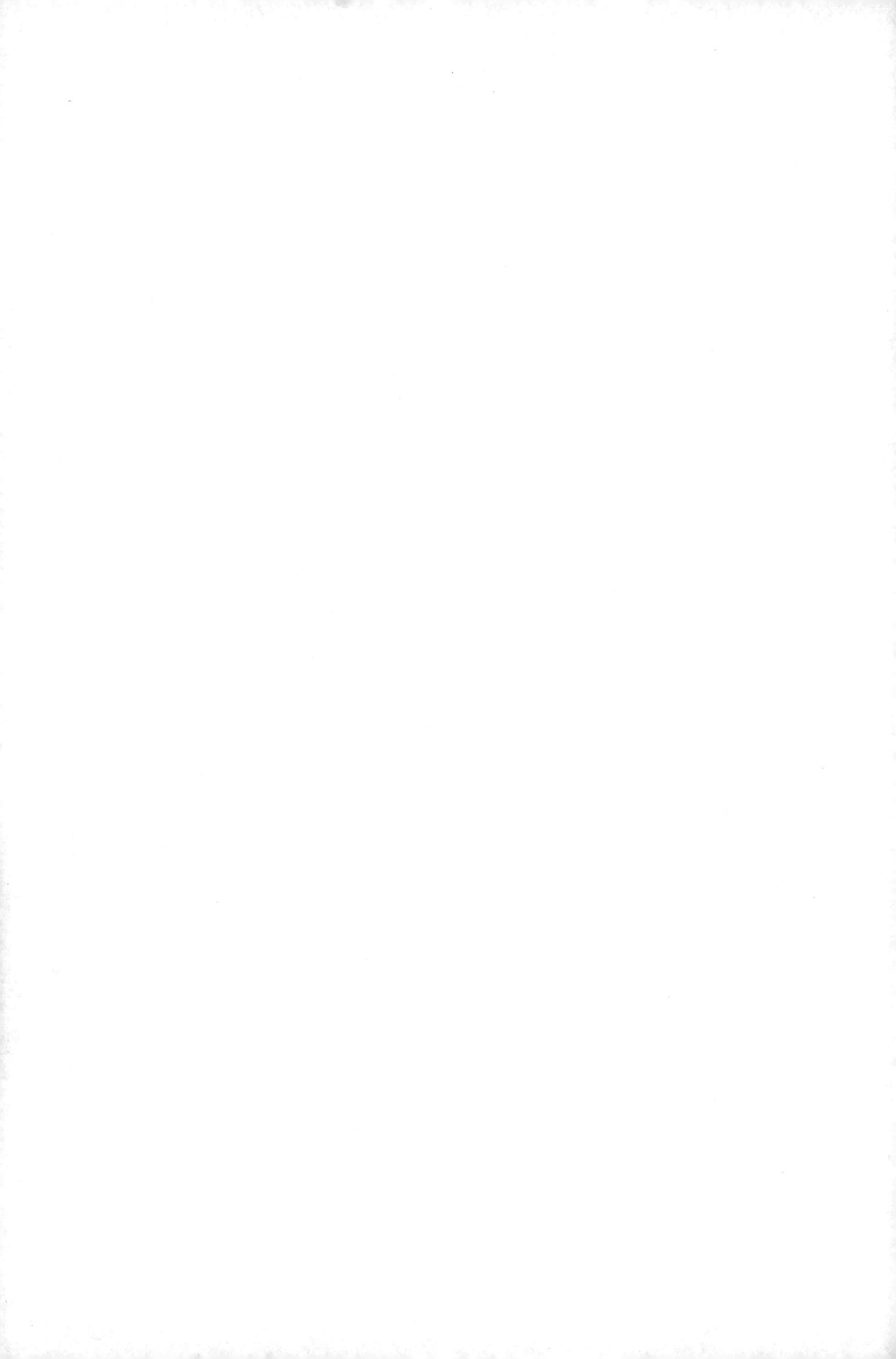

Answers to Sample Exams

Answers to Anatomy Questions

1. d	8. b	15. d	22. b	29. c
2. a	9. d	16. c	23. a	30. d
3. c	10. a	17. c	24. c	31. d
4. c	11. c	18. b	25. a	32. a
5. a	12. c	19. c	26. b	33. c
6. d	13. a	20. b	27. b	34. a
7. c	14. b	21. d	28. b	35. d

Answers to Biochemistry Questions

1. d	8. b	15. c	22. b	29. a
2. d	9. d	16. b	23. d	30. c
3. b	10. a	17. b	24. b	31. b
4. c	11. c	18. d	25. a	32. b
5. a	12. c	19. b	26. d	33. d
6. c	13. d	20. c	27. b	
7. b	14. a	21. d	28. c	

Answers to Pathology Questions

1. a	6. a	11. b	16. a	21. d
2. a	7. d	12. b	17. d	22. a
3. b	8. c	13. c	18. a	23. c
4. c	9. b	14. a	19. c	24. a
5. d	10. d	15. b	20. d	25. a

26. d	28. c	30. b	32. b	34. b
27. c	29. b	31. d	33. a	35. d

Answers to Physiology Questions

1. d	8. d	15. c	22. b	29. b
2. a	9. b	16. d	23. d	30. a
3. a	10. b	17. a	24. d	31. a
4. c	11. a	18. b	25. a	32. b
5. a	12. c	19. a	26. b	
6. b	13. b	20. a	27. c	
7. b	14. b	21. d	28. b	

Answers to Microbiology Questions

1. a	8. d	14. b	20. b	26. a
2. a	9. b	15. d	21. b	27. c
3. b	10. d	16. a	22. b	28. a
4. c	11. b	17. b	23. a	29. a
5. c	12. a	18. a	24. c	30. c
6. a	13. d	19. c	25. d	31. a
7. c				

Sources

Bonow RO, Mann DL, Zipes DP, Libby P, Braunwald E (2011) *Braunwald's Heart Disease: A Textbook Of Cardiovascular Medicine 9th ed* (Elsevier Saunders: Philadelphia, PA).

Bope ET, Kellerman RD, Rakel RE (2010) *Conn's Current Therapy* (Elsevier Saunders: Philadelphia, PA).

Bradley WG, Daroff RB, Fenichel GM, Jankovic J (2007) *Neurology in Clinical Practice 5th Ed* (Butterworth-Heinemann: Philadelphia, PA).

DeLee JC, Drez D, Millar MD (2008) *DeLee and Drez's Orthopaedic Sports Medicine* (Elsevier Saunders: Philadelphia, PA).

Feldman M, Friedman LS, Brandt LJ (2010) *Sleisenger and Fordran's Gastrointestinal and Liver Disease: Pathophysiology, Diagnosis, Management 9th Ed* (Elsevier Saunders: Philadelphia, PA).

Hoffman R, Furie B, McGlave P, et al. (2008) *Hematology: Basic Principles and Practice 5th Ed* (Churchill Livingstone: Philadelphia, PA).

Kumar V, Abbas AK, Fausto N, Aster J (2009) *Robbins and Cotran Pathologic Basis of Disease, Professional Edition, 8th Ed* (Saunders: Philadelphia, PA).

Nussey S, Whitehead S (2001) *Endrocrinology: An Integrated Approach* (BIOS Scientific Publishers Ltd: Oxford, UK).

Townsend CM, Beauchamp RD, Evers BM, Mattox KL (2008) *Sabiston Textbook of Surgery 18th Ed* (Saunders: Philadelphia, PA).